Storytelling from a Psychotherapy Perspective

Bringing together a fusion of psychology, storytelling, and feminism, *Storytelling from a Psychotherapy Perspective* presents a humorous yet highly practical anthology of traditional stories with psychological truths hidden within their fabric for mental health practitioners to draw upon in their work with clients. Readers are encouraged to draw from the well of soulful wisdom and keen insight enshrined in traditional tales and will gain a stronger understanding of the unique power of stories to create safe spaces to explore difficult personal experiences.

Written by an author with the unique dual experience of psychotherapy practice and professional storytelling, this book presents a collection of 50 traditional tales. Drawing from the metaphor of paintings in an exhibition, stories are grouped into Rooms and accompanied by psychological reflections, functioning similarly to a published catalogue. The tales are categorised into the following sections:

- Bawdy Tales
- Beastly Tales
- Transpersonal Tales
- Tales of Soul
- Original Stories
- Stories with Children

A unique contribution to therapeutic storytelling literature, this will be an essential read for both trainee and more seasoned practitioners alike working within the fields of psychotherapy, counselling, psychology and mental health coaching, and therapeutic storytelling.

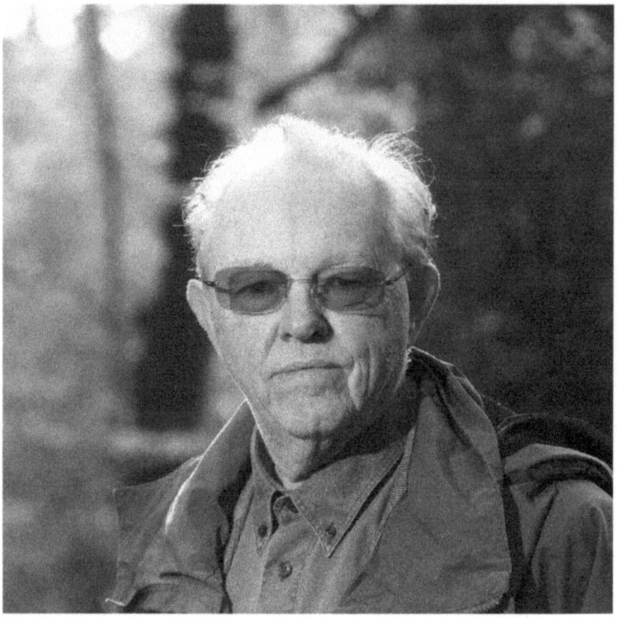

David England is a registered psychotherapist with over 25 years of experience, an author and a professional storyteller. His previously published works include *Soulfulness: The Marriage of Shamanic and Contemporary Psychology* (2017).

Storytelling from a Psychotherapy Perspective

Bawdy and Beastly Tales

David England

Routledge
Taylor & Francis Group
LONDON AND NEW YORK

Designed cover image: Jo Lowes © PufferFishPressUK

First published 2027
by Routledge
4 Park Square, Milton Park, Abingdon, Oxon OX14 4RN

and by Routledge
605 Third Avenue, New York, NY 10158

Routledge is an imprint of the Taylor & Francis Group, an informa business

British Library Cataloguing-in-Publication Data
A catalogue record for this book is available from the British Library

Library of Congress Cataloging-in-Publication Data
Names: England, David (Storyteller) author
Title: Storytelling from a psychotherapy perspective : bawdy and beastly tales / David England.
Description: Abingdon, Oxon ; New York, NY : Routledge, 2026. |
Includes bibliographical references and index. |
Identifiers: LCCN 2025053200 (print) | LCCN 2025053201 (ebook) |
ISBN 9781041195696 hbk | ISBN 9781041195689 pbk | ISBN 9781003712329 ebk
Subjects: LCSH: Narrative therapy | Psychoanalysis and fairy tales
Classification: LCC RC489.S74 E54 2026 (print) | LCC RC489.S74 (ebook)
LC record available at https://lccn.loc.gov/2025053200
LC ebook record available at https://lccn.loc.gov/2025053201

ISBN: 978-1-041-19569-6 (hbk)
ISBN: 978-1-041-19568-9 (pbk)
ISBN: 978-1-003-71232-9 (ebk)

DOI: 10.4324/9781003712329

Typeset in Times New Roman
by Newgen Publishing UK

I am pleased to dedicate this book to all my psychotherapy clients, who have taught me so much about how to do my work.

Contents

Acknowledgements *xi*
About the Author *xii*
Hawk *xiii*

PART I
Catalogue **1**

1 Preface 3
Intention 3
How You Might Use This Book 5
Introduction to the Collection 6
The Healing Power of Storytelling 7
Layout of the Book 9

2 Catalogue of Stories in the Collection 11
Bawdy Tales Room 11
Beastly Tales Room 12
Transpersonal Tales Room 12
Tales of Soul Room 13
Original Stories Room 14
Storytelling With Children Room 15

3 A Portrait of Soul 18
What I Mean by 'Soul' 18
The Dynamic Portrayal of Soul 18
The Four Elements 20
The Aspects of Being Human 21
The Gifts of Being Human 21
The Journey of Soulmaking 30

Sexuality: Consciousness and Will 35
Songs of Being Human 36

4 Storytelling as a Healing Art 38
Soul and Soulmaking 38
Soul and Imagination 38
The Sin Against the Imagination 39
A New Gestalt: A New Way of Experiencing Ourselves 39
Reality and Imagination 39
Stories State Existential Dilemmas 40
The Resonance of a Story 42
The Story As Container 43
Therapeutic Storywriting: Writing One's Own Story 44

PART II
Rooms **47**

5 Bawdy Tales Room 49
Psychological and Egalitarian Reflection 49
The Crane's Leg 50
The Laydys of the Towne 54
Demeter and Persephone 59
Defiant Saxon Queens 63
Cynethryth Queen of the Mercians 64
Queen Emma's Ordeal By Fire 67
The Abbess' Coif 72
Sir Gawain and the Green Knight 77
Pearl of Wisdom 86

6 Beastly Tales Room 92
The Unsworth Dragon 93
King Gaarge and the Dragon 98
Mr Fox 103
The Dun Cow of Parlick 108
The Great Hairy Toe 114
Lady Sybil and the Milk White Doe 118
The Witches of Windsor 122

7 Beastly Tales Annex: 'Witches' 129
Egalitarian and Scientific Reflection 129

8 Transpersonal Tales Room 131
The Work That Reconnects 131
Tales for the Great Turning 132
Psychological Reflection on These Transpersonal Tales 132
Dream Dilemma 133
The Three Golden Hairs 134
Tiddalik the Frog: In the Dreamtime 136
The King and the Oak 139
Iris—Rainbow Goddess 141
The Tiger and the Strawberry 143
A Woman Made of Salt: A Traditional Spiritual Story 145
My Lord Bag of Rice 146
The Young Man, the Lion, and the Yellow-Flowered Storm-Cloud Tree 151

9 Tales of Soul Room 154
Vasilisa and Baba Yaga 155
The Horse of Power 163
Sir Gawain and the Loathly Lady 170
Telling Tales 176
The Feeling In Her Bones 177
The Juniper Tree 181
Saint Corentin and the Golden Fish 186

10 Original Stories Room 191
Traveller's Tales 191
The Man On the Up Escalator—A Christmas Story 192
The Girl With Green Hair 194
At the Dove At Chiswick 196
In Burlington Arcade 197
Dreaming of Place 199
Dark Night of the Soul 200
Once Upon A Time the Land Rejoiced As A Princess Was Born 203

11 Storytelling With Children Room 207
The Creative Power of Storytelling With Children 208
The Three Spinners 211
Getting Rid of the Mice 214
The Hat Seller 216
The Golden Bowl 218
Pinonçita, The Very Little Girl 220
The Crystal Ball 223
The Well of the World's End 227
The Greatest Gift 231
The Naming of Cuchullin 234

12 Ending: The Meaning of Life 237

13 Sting in the Tale 239

Index *240*

Acknowledgements

I am pleased to acknowledge Susannah Frearson, Routledge Publisher, for her willingness to engage in dialogue with me and for her astute feedback, which served to make the book fit for publication by Routledge.

I am pleased to acknowledge Routledge Editor Lauren Redhead and Editorial Assistant Tanishka Luhia for their attentiveness and wise counsel throughout the editing process, and Charmitha Ashok, Project Manager of production, for patiently shepherding the book to market.

I am pleased to acknowledge my Readers, Susan Holliday, Wendy Smit, and Ed England, for their unfailing support and their incisive and gracious feedback during the writing of this book.

About the Author

I am a psychotherapist and writer. As a psychotherapist, I am a novice of 25 years standing. As a writer, I have several previously published articles and books, principally 'Soulfulness' (Routledge 2017). It goes without saying, I am also a storyteller.

Psychotherapy, writing, and storytelling is what I choose to do. It is not who I am.

This is who I am. I am imaginative and intuitive, original in my thoughts. I believe in the power of language, spoken and written, to create meaningful connection. I value love, friendship, clarity, and authenticity. My favourite word is 'grace'. I take no credit for such qualities and values; they come by grace from a source deep within. They are the guiding principles of my life and the legacy I am here to pass on to others.

Hawk

The image on the book's cover is a Hawk silhouetted
against a hazy sun.
This Hawk image symbolises the Transpersonal Journey
of the Soul:
Wind beneath its wings.
Intent on touching the stars,
Hawk's eyes scan the earth.
The essence of the Transpersonal Journey distilled
into 14 words.
Inviting reflection.

Part I

Catalogue

An art exhibition has a catalogue to read and exhibition rooms to browse in.

Like an art exhibition, this book has a Catalogue to explain the book and Rooms to exhibit the stories.

The Catalogue includes:

Preface: states the book's intention, discusses how reader and writer might relate, how psychological truths lie hidden within the fabric of traditional tales, how the reader might use the book, provides an introduction to traditional tales and the healing power of stories, describes the layout of the book, and introduces the categories of Rooms in which the stories are contained.

The book aims to inspire counsellors, psychotherapists, coaches, and therapeutic storytellers to draw upon the deep well of soulful wisdom and keen insight enshrined in traditional tales.

Catalogue of Stories in the Collection: shows the Rooms and the stories they contain. For each story, there is a brief description designed to lure the reader into perusing it. This is a browsing book. From the Catalogue of Stories, the reader can choose a Room to browse in or a story to peruse.

A Portrait of Soul: sets out for the therapist the core psychology upon which the book is based, including a real-time representation of a human Soul and the growth of their consciousness and will throughout life.

Storytelling as a Healing Art: presents the writer's perception of the relationship between storytelling and psychology, founded upon the maxim, the story is the healer.

DOI: 10.4324/9781003712329-1

Preface

Bawdy and Beastly Tales is a colourful, living tapestry with scenes of life woven into a pattern of light and dark shades to illumine your therapy space.

Intention

Storytelling from a Psychotherapy Perspective: Bawdy and Beastly Tales is a psychology book from cover to cover. Yet, it is a funny kind of psychology book. *Bawdy and Beastly Tales* is a fusion and rich profusion of psychology, storytelling, and feminism, with a dollop of autobiography and a pinch of humour. Being a psychotherapist and a storyteller, *Bawdy and Beastly Tales* is a collection of traditional tales, as retold by me, set within a psychological framework.

My intention in writing *Bawdy and Beastly Tales* is to inspire counsellors, psychotherapists, coaches, and therapeutic storytellers to draw upon the deep well of soulful wisdom and keen insight enshrined in traditional tales and to convey the unique power of stories to illuminate corners of otherwise unspeakable darkness. This book makes available a wealth of intriguing, magical, comical, and enchanting tales to illustrate the psychotherapeutic power of imagination.

The Book as a Dialogue

I see this book as a kind of dialogue between writer and reader. As writer, I have an unqualified regard for the reader, and respect their right to their views, however much they may differ from mine. I shall address you throughout in the second person singular. I shall share with you the thoughts arising for me from the stories and invite you in reply to reflect on what they mean for you. I shall strive never to express my views in an assertive manner. I invite you to be a party to this dialogue.

"Purveyors of Deep Insight"

I go along with Bruno Bettelheim, in his book *The Uses of Enchantment* (1976), who recognises psychological truths hidden within the fabric of traditional tales.

DOI: 10.4324/9781003712329-2

He describes these tales as "the purveyors of deep insight that have sustained mankind through the long vicissitudes of its existence," tales that characteristically "state an existential dilemma briefly and pointedly," and "represent in imaginative form what the process of healthy human development consists of."

Bawdy and Beastly Tales is a collection of 50 traditional tales. They are grouped into Rooms, like paintings in an exhibition. What binds together an exhibition of paintings is the published Catalogue, and alongside each Canvas is a brief description. What binds together this collection of stories is *A Portrait of Soul*, the book's core psychology, and alongside each 'Canvas' are psychological reflections drawing on *A Portrait of Soul*.

Psychological Reflections

Throughout the book are my preambles and interjections. My preambles are the autobiographical element of the book. Each preamble is a candid note or anecdote expressing my relationship with the story that follows. Interjections are my way of putting in a personal word in the middle of a story. Preambles are shown in boxes. Interjections are shown in italics within curly brackets.

Each story in the collection is self-contained, including, with variations: my preamble, a synopsis, the story, its sources—where I found inspiration to write my version of the story—and accompanying psychological reflections.

The psychological reflections comprise:

Your Psychological Reflections. Suggestions to assist you, the reader, to strengthen your psychological grasp of the story.

My Psychological Reflections. I have needed to tread a fine line between offering my reflections and giving an interpretation, because it is not up to the teller, it is up to the hearer or reader, to decide what they take from a story.

Egalitarian Reflections.

The ill treatment of women is a common feature of traditional stories, and because the denial of women's rights and oppression and violence towards women is a deep concern for me, I draw this out in my reflections.

The more I know about women the less I claim to understand. The more I know about women the higher is my regard. Gloria Steinem, author of *My Life on the Road* (2015), is attributed with the quotation, "A feminist is anyone who recognizes the equality and full humanity of women and men." I have always recognised this, so it feels natural to call myself a feminist writer, along with Alexander Pope, Thomas Hardy, and Grayson Perry.

How You Might Use This Book

Bawdy and Beastly Tales offers an immersive, imaginative experience in story, a vista over rich, deep, fertile lands, to support you in your psychotherapeutic professional work.

There are 50 separate stories in the Collection. The Rooms and stories are listed and introduced in the *Catalogue of Stories* below. Each time you pick up the book, you have a choice. You may read the book straight through. Or, like an art exhibition, you may choose a Room and go there to browse. Or you may select a particular tale to peruse.

Reading a psychology book can be for me largely an intellectual exercise, what I am *learning*. Attending an art exhibition, on the other hand, is to *experience* the paintings, the feelings and visceral senses, thoughts, and intuitions which they evoke, and this is the inspiration I can take away and which can remain with me, my *Soul*[1] *experience.*

Reading a Story

I invite you to experience a story, the feelings and visceral senses, thoughts, images, and intuitions which the story evokes, whilst letting your Soul experience inform your appreciation of its underlying psychology. In other words, to find a creative space between Soul experience and psychological discovery.

Every story has three main elements: action, description, emotion. Be aware of these elements and dig down further. Who are the characters in the story? Observe them like they are clients in your therapy room or group. What are their personalities? What are the dynamics between them? What are your feelings about them, your responses and reactions? Where do your sympathies lie? To what degree would you like them in your therapy room? What is the mood of the story?

In therapy, there comes a turning point, so what is the turning point in the story?

Reflect on the story after reading it. What is its emotional impact? Then, read the psychological reflections, read the story again. What do you perceive about psychological depth in the story?

Gender Diversity

Gender identities, demonstrating a diversity of expression beyond the binary man/woman understanding of gender, is a reality that has come to be recognised and acknowledged in recent times. I have not found such gender diversity present in traditional stories emerging from former times. So, where I discuss 'men' and 'women' in this book, I leave it to you to make any necessary extrapolations.

Therapeutic Storytelling

Any telling of a tale offers the promise of healing, having the power to touch the Soul, to change lives. My maxim regarding the healing power of stories is, "The story is the healer." This is discussed in depth in the section *Storytelling as a Healing Art*. Each of the stories in the Collection is available for retelling. Just, thoroughly take in the tale and tell it in your own way.

If you plan to tell stories from this Collection in a therapeutic setting, here are my suggestions:

Select the stories that fit your setting, maybe a group of children, adolescents, or adults, or a more specialist group, maybe elderly people, or grieving children, families, or adults.

Thoroughly read, reread, take in the stories and accompanying reflections.

Reflect on each story. What do I take from it? What does it mean for me? What therapeutic meaning has it for me.

Map out or write the story as you now perceive it, as appropriate for your setting.

In addition, here are two well-respected books on therapeutic storytelling:

Helping Children Cope with Loss and Change by Amanda Seyderhelm.

Routledge International Handbook of Therapeutic Stories and Storytelling, edited by Clive Holmwood, Sue Jennings, Sharon Jacksties.

Introduction to the Collection

This section explains the core concept underlying *Bawdy and Beastly Tales* within the living tradition of storytelling.

Telling Tales: The Book's Core Concept

Traditional storytelling is a living tradition, as storytellers retell tales that have emerged from the mists of time.

I discovered traditional tales during my training in psychosynthesis psychotherapy, a short time before I wrote my MA thesis. It struck me that many folk tales have a psychological resonance, so this became the core concept underlying the thesis, as well as suggesting a title with a dual meaning, *Telling Tales*.

I have applied the same idea, traditional tales having a psychological resonance, as the core concept underlying *Bawdy and Beastly Tales*.

Storytelling: a Living Tradition

Storytelling is a millennia-spanning, world-spanning oral tradition, whenever and wherever people tell tales to other people.

A traditional tale is told and retold down the generations, with each storyteller telling the tale in their own way, their own individual perception of the story.

Another way of passing stories on to new generations is through collections, the best known collection of stories being Grimm's Fairy Tales. The finest and most extensive collection is from The History Press, a book of Folk Tales for every county in the UK, written not by collectors but by practising storytellers, giving these books the ring of authenticity.

What this means is that, by passing on a traditional tale, by word or by print, the psychological truths hidden within its fabric are passed on as well.

Creation Myth of the San People

From the earliest times, with our capacity to think, we have reflected about the world we see about us. Then something wonderful happens, over time there emerge myths and tales regarding observable natural phenomena and the powers that control them, about gods and about the creation of the world. Every ancient community conceived its own creation myth to describe the earliest beginnings of the world. The *List of Creation Myths*[2] on the Wikipedia website lists and links to many creation myths, which amazingly are still told today by storytellers worldwide. Each creation myth has been told and retold through countless generations, right down to the present day.

The San people of the Kalahari Desert are the oldest community of people in the world, with 140,000 years of history. Here is their creation myth, the oldest story in the world.

> Before time was, before land emerges from the primordial waters encircling the earth, Bee bears Mantis, between her slender legs, above the endless sea, searching a place to set Mantis down. All Bee sees is ceaseless sea, coming closer as her wings exhaust. Bee espies a flower floating on the swell, its petals reaching out like welcoming arms. She places Mantis softly on the flower. She stings Mantis, planting a seed in Mantis' body. Bee dies. The seed grows to become the first human being. So begins Mantis, the maker of fire, the keeper of the hearth.

Deceptively simple, this short and ancient creation myth is full of meaning; for me, Bee is the first cause, the creator. Bee sacrifices her life for her creation, itself a not unfamiliar theme. Here, at the beginning of creation, the myth introduces the cycle of death and birth, Bee sacrificing her life so that something more, the human race, shall be brought to birth.

The Healing Power of Storytelling

Telling tales has the power to inspire, to touch the Soul, and thereby to change lives, and at its heart the power is in the quality of relationship between teller and listeners. Here's an illustration.

The Girl Who Loved to Dance

I am at Dance Camp East as resident storyteller. One of the organisers tells me her story,

> "As a child, I loved to dance. People admired my dancing, so more and more I danced for them rather than for myself. One day, I lost my feet. Ever since, I have been unable to dance."

She asks me to write her story, so that, as I tell her story, with musical accompaniment, she can dance again.

I take myself off to a café for a couple of hours and write, *The Girl Who Loved to Dance*. Later, I tell the story as she dances, for herself, the first time since she was a child. Here is the story, *The Girl Who Loved to Dance*:

Once upon a time, there was a girl who loved to dance.

All admired her dancing. So, she danced to be admired.

One day, as she danced, she lost her feet. She fell to the ground. When she rose, her movements were clumsy, without grace.

She looked down. She saw she had really lost her feet. She saw her knees and calves, but no feet.

Without feet the girl could no longer dance. She was no longer admired. She felt unseen.

She hid herself in the forest. The gloom of the forest reflected her mood; the heavy boughs the sorrow in her heart.

One day, she was captivated by a harebell:

She lost herself in its pliant dance in the gentle morning breeze.

She lost herself in the still dance of the hovering kestrel. The swift dance of the swallow.

She lost herself in the slow dance of old oaks. The solemn swaying of beech.

She lost herself in the scurrying dance of beetles in rotting timber. The intent dance of ants.

She lost herself in the shy dance of the graceful fallow deer.

She lost herself in the predatory circle dance of wolves.

One day, she found her feet. She began to dance. In the dance she found herself:

She found the dance of harebell and bluebell.

She found the dance of kestrel and swallow.

She found the dance of oak and beech.

She found the dance of beetle and ant.

She found the desperate dance of fallow deer and wolf.

Returning, she danced the wild dance of the forest. The wild life of the forest.

The woman who loves to dance.

Next Dance Camp East, I meet a woman in the Wellbeing Tent who wants to tell stories but is too scared. I tell her about *The Girl Who Loved to Dance*. The next day she is excited to tell me how she had told the story the previous evening in her campfire circle. That evening, I had been booked to tell tales in the same campfire circle, and after the telling a woman tells me her story,

> "Early this year, I lost the use of my legs. I couldn't walk. I have learnt to walk again. I have come to the Dance Camp in the hope of dancing again. Last evening, something amazing happened. A woman in my campfire circle told a story about a girl who lost her feet and couldn't dance, then found her feet again, and she danced. Today, after listening to the story, I found my feet and I danced again."

The woman doesn't know that the story has gone round and back to me, inspiring all three of us and changing our lives. The healing power of storytelling.

Layout of the Book

Following the 'art exhibition' metaphor, *Bawdy and Beastly Tales* consists of a Catalogue and Rooms for the exhibits.

Catalogue

The Catalogue comprises the present Preface and a further three sections:

Catalogue of Stories in the Collection: This section lists the Rooms and the Stories within them and provides a synopsis of each story, designed to lure you into perusing it.

A Portrait of Soul: This section sets out the core psychology upon which the book is based. The subsection *The Dynamic Portrayal of Soul,* founded on the Native American Medicine Wheel, provides for therapists a real-time representation of a whole person, their constituent elements, how these interrelate, how energy is deployed, how the person changes in time. The subsection *The Journey of Soulmaking* describes the expansion of a person's consciousness and will in three phases: Pre-personal, Personal, and Transpersonal. References to *A Portrait of Soul* throughout the Psychological Reflections are indicated by underlining.

Storytelling as a Healing Art: This section presents my perception of the relationship between storytelling and psychology, my appreciation of how stories have a healing power, expressed in the maxim, 'The story is the healer'.

Rooms

There are six exhibition Rooms:

Bawdy Tales. On rare occasions, I have been allowed the ultimate privilege that a man can be afforded: to sit in on women's talk, so fast and fluid, so effortlessly comic, so sublimely bawdy. I hope these tales exude something of the same spirit. To my mind and heart, the traditional tales in this section are an acknowledgement of the skilful will, moral strength, incisive wit, and acute inner wisdom possessed by women and embodied in women's sexuality.

Beastly Tales. From earliest times, beasts have burrowed into the souls of human beings, nesting, nestling, and roosting until emerging in ancient tales as shape-shifting creatures, creatures of romance, creatures of fear and fun, creatures of wonder, creatures of nightmare—a shadow of the real-life horror spewing from the tormented mind of man.

Transpersonal Tales. The transpersonal goes beyond a person's capacity for self-reflection to a sense of intimate self-reflexive consciousness, of other human beings, of other creatures, of the world of nature, of the world we live in.

Tales of Soul is a set of stories with a distinct psychological context, tales of mind, heart, and soul, including three explicitly psychological stories that I included in my MA thesis, which was a reflection on the relationship between traditional stories and psychological sufferings.

Original Stories are mainly *Traveller's Tales* that I wrote before I discovered psychosynthesis psychology, observation pieces that show some aptitude for qualities that subsequently serve me as a therapist.

Storytelling with Children. These tales illustrate the creative power of storytelling with children, as well as illustrating my interactive style of storytelling with children. Throughout the book, a story suitable for telling to children or adolescents is indicated beneath its title.

Notes

1 I discuss 'Soul' in the *A Portrait of Soul* section.
2 https://en.wikipedia.org/wiki/List_of_creation_myths

Bibliography

Bettelheim, Bruno (1989) *The Uses of Enchantment*, Vintage.
Holmwood, Clive, Jennings, Sue, and Jacksties, Sharon (Eds) (1922) *Routledge International Handbook of Therapeutic Stories and Storytelling*, Routledge.
Seyderhelm, Amanda (2019) *Helping Children Cope with Loss and Change: A Guide for Professionals and Parents*, Routledge.
Steinem, Gloria (2015) *My Life on the Road*, Random House.
Wikipedia Website, *List of Creation Myths*.

Catalogue of Stories in the Collection

This Catalogue lists the Rooms and the Stories within them, and provides a synopsis of each story, designed to lure you into perusing it, and provides Page Numbers for Stories in the Collection.
There are also two stories in the Preface:
Creation Myth of the San People
The Girl Who Loved to Dance

Bawdy Tales Room

The Crane's Leg: A Tuscan noble's hawks bring down a plump crane. The pastry cook entices the cook into sharing a thigh with her. The Tuscan noble plans revenge and humiliation. How does a mere pastry cook use her wit and wisdom to better the noble?

The Laydys of the Towne: A contemporary account of how the alluring laydys enact an amorous approach to ending the 1715 Jacobite rebellion. What does the tale tell of skilful will and moral strength in women?

Demeter and Persephone: Hades carries off Persephone to be Queen of the Underworld, to Demeter's chagrin. How do Baubo's bawdy jokes touch Demeter's Soul and restore her Spirit so as to trounce Hades?

Cynethryth Queen of the Mercians: Cynethryth wields her wiles upon King Offa to become Queen of Mercia. With her sharp wits and wicked nature, she single-handedly adds the Kingdom of East Anglia to their domains. Despite all, could this be a redemptive tale?

Queen Emma's Ordeal By Fire: To maintain her queenship, after King Cnut had successfully invaded her land, Queen Emma adroitly seduces Cnut into marriage. How can it be that this proves a successful union?

The Abbess' Coif: To avoid a marriage dowry, a nobleman consigns his daughter to a religious order of nuns. Far from submissively embracing her confinement, she embraces a young gallant. How does she assert her independence and self-determination?

Sir Gawain and the Green Knight: Sir Gawain accepts a challenge from the Green Knight to exchange blow for blow, at the neck. Heading to a northern castle, he

DOI: 10.4324/9781003712329-3

is enchanted by its lady, who engages him in courtly love, before the axe falls. What can we learn of courtly love?

Pearl of Wisdom: A king with bizarre and unimaginable sexual fantasies seeks to select a wife with whom to fulfil his desires. This voluptuous woman is intent rather in fulfilling his, and her own, deepest yearnings. What's conveyed of woman's relational sexuality?

Beastly Tales Room

The Unsworth Dragon: For generations, a terrible dragon has burst from its lair and ravaged the surrounding country, venting rage and retribution on womankind. With a dragon invulnerable to bullets, how can Thomas Unsworth end his family's generational trauma?

King Gaarge and the Dragon: A milkmaid finds an earthworm on her pillow. Odd? Keeps it as a pet! It grows into a dragon with a taste for milk and maidens. They feed it six pails of milk a day plus a maiden chosen by lot, until King Gaarge canters up. Could Draca be the serpent inside?

Mr Fox: Before marrying enigmatic Mr Fox, Lady Mary, young and fair, seeks his castle home in the deepest, darkest part of the forest, there to discover his deepest, darkest secret. Hasn't Lady Mary every reason to mistrust Mr Fox, his name alone?

The Dun Cow of Parlick: At a time of famine, a dun cow appears with an abundant supply of milk for the villagers, just as an old hag appears to provide them with ceramic milking pots. So, why then does she use a sieve to drain the dun cow dry of the villagers milk?

The Great Hairy Toe: A scruffy old women foraging for mushrooms finds a great hairy toe. She cooks and eats it. Ugh! In the night a distant voice cries, I want my great hairy toe. As the voice gets closer, she hides beneath her narrow bed. Can there be a happy ending?

Lady Sybil and the Milk White Doe: Lady Sybil loves to roam the wide moor, learning its secret lore. Lord William fears she'll be accused of witchcraft. Guided by a wise-woman with a game leg, he looses hounds in pursuit of a milk white doe. Who's the craggy old bitch with a game hind leg, outpacing the rest, gently holding the doe's leg in her jaws?

The Witches of Windsor: In Elizabethan Windsor, four impoverished old wise-women, accused of witchcraft by Richard Galis, are arrested and imprisoned, one of them making a detailed fictitious confession in Richard Galis' presence, and then hanged. Why do they sing a song of thanksgiving all the way to the scaffold?

Transpersonal Tales Room

Dream Dilemma: A man dreams he is a butterfly, freeing himself from the chrysalis, opening his wings, a beautiful pattern of red and orange, flecked with white and yellow. He is enthralled. Waking, he ponders, "Am I a man dreaming he's a butterfly, or a butterfly, dreaming I'm a man?" What do you ponder?

The Three Golden Hairs: A frail old man makes painful progress through the forest. Reaching a cottage, an old woman gathers him up, gently holds him as he becomes by dawn a beautiful young child, and plucks three of his golden hairs. Giving her a warm smile, he leaps into the sky, the bright sun. What can renew your energy?

Tiddalik the Frog: In the Dreamtime: In the time before time, a very fat frog swallows all the water in the world. The earth is parched, plants die. Other animals are gasping; they plan to make the frog laugh, so he'll squirt out all the water to fill the rivers, streams, and pools. How might laughter equip us with the harmony to face shared challenges?

The King and the Oak: Near a sacred grove, watched over by Demeter, there lives a mighty king, who decides to chop down the grove to build a palace, despite Demeter's warning that drought and hunger would follow. Will the sacred grove remain forever barren?

Iris—Rainbow Goddess: Iris, she alone of all the gods, rides the rainbow. Iris sails her chariot, drawn by a pair of dazzling peacocks, casting her radiant rainbow where she will. The Rainbow Goddess plays wherever she lets the light of sun or moon illuminate the misty clouds and waterfalls. Shall she forever succour humankind?

The Tiger and the Strawberry: To illustrate the elusive nature of human happiness, Buddha narrated the vivid story of a man who, while roaming in the forest, was discovered and hotly pursued by a tiger. How shall we savour the sublime second simply for itself?

A Woman Made of Salt: A Traditional Spiritual Story: A woman made of salt lives beside the Great Ocean, the eighth ocean of the world. As time passes, she feels herself drawn more and more to the Great Ocean, longs to plumb its depths, to know its span. Shall she forever savour the sublime second?

My Lord Bag of Rice: A warrior, servant of the sun god, gathers his scimitars, a great bow, and all his courage, to set off on a quest to right wrongs. He faces a fearsome dragon, which turns out to be a grieving old man, the Dragon King in the guise of a dragon. The Dragon King is beset by a horrific beast, who has grown fat on the bodies and souls of his sons and daughters, a centipede. "A centipede!" I hear you cry.

The Young Man, the Lion, and the Yellow-Flowered Storm-Cloud Tree: A young man lies down to rest beside a waterhole, later visited by a thirsty lion. When he sees the young man weeping with fear, the thirsty lion licks the tears from his cheeks. This proves fatal for them both. How challenging do you find this tale?

Tales of Soul Room

Vasilisa and Baba Yaga: The story follows a life's journey: a child at mother's deathbed; a subdued childhood spent with a callous and demanding mother and bullying sisters; her life in the forest, overcoming her fears to move forward;

finding a wise-woman whom she can respect and be willing to be guided by. How would you portray your Journey of Soulmaking?

The Horse of Power: A young archer finds a firebird's golden feather as he rides through the forest on the Horse of Power, who cautions him: Leave the feather where it lies, else you will learn the meaning of fear. How might you have felt the lure of temptation?

Sir Gawain and the Loathly Lady: The Loathly Lady Ragnell imagines how to wed Gawain: move deliberately; entrap King Arthur; get Gawain's consent to an unwelcome alliance; most difficult of all, make sure Gawain respects her enough to leave her the crucial decision. What may be your experience of redemption found in relationship?

The Feeling In Her Bones: A father throws his daughter over a cliff into the sea. Fish eat her flesh, till nought remains but the feeling in her bones. A sailor fishes her out. Caught up in his line, she follows him home. He's in for a shock he'll never regret. What was it like for you, the first time you asserted your personal will?

The Juniper Tree: A mother has a moment of joy at her son's birth, then she dies. The stepmother knocks his block off, blaming her daughter, who buries his bones beneath the juniper tree, whence he emerges as a beautiful bird, Keewitt, keewitt. What a fine bird am I. To what extent, and in what way, does this tale strike a chord?

Saint Corentin and the Golden Fish: During his Lenten fast, desire for nourishment fills the Friar's aching body and soul. He sees, in the spring pool, a golden fish. He is tormented—eats the fish—is conscience stricken—throws the bones in the pool. Next day the fish is swimming in the pool, setting the pattern for his Lenten spiritual practice. What do 'crisis of meaning' and 'soulmaking' mean for you?

Original Stories Room

The Man On the Up Escalator—A Christmas Story: Hundreds of us ride the escalators, with our dark thoughts of Christmas future. One man, sober and grey, wears a Father Christmas hat. He creates a bow wave of curiosity and humour. He lifts our spirits, lightens our Christmas darkness.

This tale invites you to reflect on your quality of humour.

The Girl With Green Hair: On the Piccadilly Line into London, the girl sits next to me, reading King Lear for A level. She turns and asks me, "What's fumitory?" We commence a meaningful talk about death.

This tale invites you to reflect on your quality of empathy.

At the Dove At Chiswick: Pint in hand on the veranda of The Dove at Chiswick, overlooking the Thames, I follow an incautious impulse to challenge a Hurrah Henry's offensive remark about Liverpool.

This tale invites you to reflect on your quality of courage.

In Burlington Arcade: Browsing the antique shops of Burlington Arcade, I am addressed by a stranger who seems to know me and lots about me, putting me off my guard, a consummate professional.

This tale invites you to reflect on how easy it is to be taken in.

Dreaming of Place: At the field brow, just a circle of grass of darker shade and lusher texture than the surrounding field, like a fairy circle I think. Then the dream begins.

This tale invites you to reflect on your quality of imagination.

Dark Night of the Soul: I read this book in the Castle pub garden. A gang of lads is at a nearby table, their attention flitting about, making lewd remarks. They spot me. I walk to their table slowly. All human life is here, leadership, suspicion, attentive care, courtesy, pride, tragedy.

This tale invites you to reflect on your quality of observation.

Once Upon A Time the Land Rejoiced As A Princess Was Born: Princess Veronica watches over her little brother Adam as he goes off on his Great Quest fighting dragons. He is beguiled into entering the Circles of Enchantment to face his fiercest dragon foe and is torn to pieces. Even then, she protects his spirit. What name would you give to your inner child, and why?

Storytelling With Children Room

The Three Spinners: The queen takes Rose to the palace, "If you spin all this flax you shall marry the crown prince. You shall be a princess." But Rose does not like spinning flax. How to solve the dilemma? Get the children to help.

Getting Rid of the Mice: There's just one thing marring the king's luxurious lifestyle, the palace is overrun with mice. Children suggest cats to chase out the mice. The palace is overrun with cats. Children suggest dogs to chase out the cats …. How will it end?

The Hat Seller: An old hat seller, visiting villages to sell beautiful hats, falls asleep under a mango tree. Children, howling and scratching their armpits, like a bevy of monkeys, come down from the tree, put on his hats, and go back up, making a monkey out of him. Will the old hat seller's granddaughter fare any better? Fat chance.

The Golden Bowl: King's grumpy, so Queen's grumpy, even King's dog's grumpy, everyone's grumpy. Then a present arrives, 'Give this golden bowl to the one you love the best.' King gives it to Queen, who gives it to … all round the palace, with the children's help. Now King's happy, Queen's happy … who ends up with the bowl?

Pinonçita, The Very Little Girl: A very, very little girl ventures into the field behind the house when mother's back is turned. Spurred on by the children, she has scary adventures in yucky places, so when she gets home she has grown to be a normal-sized child just like you or me. So, how'd you like to share her scary adventures?

The Crystal Ball: A young man searches for the most beautiful woman in all the world. When he finds her, after seven years, she's atop the Crystal Mountain.

He's at its foot. There's another problem: an evil and wicked sorcerer has put her under a spell, so she's the least beautiful woman in all the world. Is it all worth the effort?

The Well of the World's End: Moira is sent for water from this well by her unkind stepmother. She's given a sieve for the water. A little frog at the well tells her how to fill the sieve with water. But she must do all he asks of her all day and all night long. The frog's a bit of a pest, but it's a fairy story, so it all works out well. Does Frog sing a good song?

The Greatest Gift: A magic telescope, magic carpet, and magic lemon are all three brothers have to save the life of a far-off princess, in return for a bag of gold and the princess's hand. How will they get there? Will she be pleased to see them? Whom shall she marry?

The Naming of Cuchullin: A champion hurler, the lad's invited to blacksmith Culann's Cèilidh, but the gates are locked and the lad has to fight Culann's ferocious cur. It's a touching tale. How does the Ulster hero get his name?

Page Numbers for Stories in the Collection

Bawdy Tales Room
The Crane's Leg 11, 50–3
The Laydys of the Towne 11, 54–8
Demeter and Persephone 11, 59–62
Cynethryth Queen of the Mercians 11, 64–6
Queen Emma's Ordeal By Fire 11, 67–71
The Abbess' Coif 11, 72–6
Sir Gawain and the Green Knight 11, 77–85
Pearl of Wisdom 12, 86–90

Beastly Tales Room
The Unsworth Dragon 12, 93–7
Mr Fox 12, 103–7
The Dun Cow of Parlick 12, 108–13
The Great Hairy Toe 12, 114–7
Lady Sybil and the Milk White Doe 12, 118–21
The Witches of Windsor 12, 122–7

Transpersonal Tales Room
Dream Dilemma 12, 133
The Three Golden Hairs 13, 134–5
Tiddalik the Frog: In the Dreamtime 13, 136–8
The King and the Oak 13, 139–40
Iris—Rainbow Goddess 13, 141–2
The Tiger and the Strawberry 13, 143–4
A Woman Made of Salt:

A Traditional Spiritual Story 13, 145
My Lord Bag of Rice 13, 146–50
The Young Man, the Lion, and the
Yellow-Flowered Storm-Cloud Tree 13, 151–3

Tales of Soul Room
Vasilisa and Baba Yaga 13–4, 155–62
The Horse of Power 14, 163–9
Sir Gawain and the Loathly Lady 14, 170–5
Telling Tales 176
The Feeling In Her Bones 14, 177–80
The Juniper Tree 14, 181–5
Saint Corentin and the Golden Fish 14, 186–90

Original Stories Room
Traveller's Tales 191
The Man On the Up Escalator—A Christmas Story 14, 192–3
The Girl With Green Hair 14, 194–5
At the Dove At Chiswick 14, 196
In Burlington Arcade 15, 197–8
Dreaming of Place 15, 199
Dark Night of the Soul 15, 200–2
Once Upon A Time the Land Rejoiced
As A Princess Was Born 15, 203–6

Storytelling With Children Room
The Creative Power of Storytelling
With Children 208–10
The Three Spinners 15, 211–3
Getting Rid of the Mice 15, 214–5
The Hat Seller 15, 216–7
The Golden Bowl 15, 218–9
Pinonçita, The Very Little Girl 15, 220–2
The Crystal Ball 15–6, 223–6
The Well of the World's End 16, 227–30
The Greatest Gift 16, 231–3
The Naming of Cuchullin 16, 234–6

A Portrait of Soul

A Portrait of Soul explains the core psychology upon which the book is based. The subsection *The Dynamic Portrayal of Soul* provides for therapists a real-time representation of a whole person, their constituent elements, how these interrelate, how energy is deployed, how the person changes in time. The subsection *The Journey of Soulmaking* describes the expansion of a person's consciousness and will in three phases: Pre-personal, Personal, and Transpersonal.

We will have open heart to heart communication
when we are intimate with one another.
Harley SwiftDeer Reagan

What I Mean by 'Soul'

In this book, I use the term 'Soul'. I need to be clear what I mean by 'Soul'. In the Vasilisa and Baba Yaga story (*Tales of Soul Room*), there is a charming image: the dying mother's soul "flew from her like a white bird, soared out of the window, and was gone." In hospitals, even today, when a patient dies they open a window to let their soul fly out. A charming image, yes, but not what I mean by Soul.

I speak not about *having a Soul* but *being a Soul*. The expressive definition of 'Soul' in the Shorter Oxford Dictionary is 'animate existence'; 'animate', from Latin *animatus*, meaning 'give breath to,' 'enliven'. So, for me, Soul is the animate experience of being alive. In other words, Soul is my present, whole, lived, embodied experience of myself, my existential reality.

The Dynamic Portrayal of Soul

In my book *Soulfulness: The Marriage of Shamanic and Contemporary Psychology* (2017), I describe the Native American Medicine Wheel as "a well developed theoretical understanding of the working of the human psyche" (Chapter 1, p. 9) and "a map of the various elements of the human personality—body, feelings, mind, spirituality, and sexuality in its widest sense as the lifeforce" (Chapter 3, p. 35).

DOI: 10.4324/9781003712329-4

The Dynamic Portrayal of Soul now provides a comprehensive description of the psychotherapeutic application of the Medicine Wheel.

Held in secret within Native American culture for hundreds of years, Harley SwiftDeer Reagan (*Shamanic Wheels and Keys*, 1994, published by Deer Tribe Metis Medicine Society[1]) was authorised to make the psychospiritual wisdom of the Medicine Wheel available to the wider world. SwiftDeer called his portrayal of a human being based on the Medicine Wheel *The Four Elements*. I refer to the portrayal of a human being based on the Medicine Wheel as *The Dynamic Portrayal of Soul*.

My aim here is to remain faithful to SwiftDeer's beautifully compassionate account of *The Four Elements* and at the same time to serve the needs of therapists for a dynamic, robust, comprehensive, and realistic portrayal of a human soul.

The following two pages reproduce pages 22 and 32 from SwiftDeer's *Shamanic Wheels and Keys,* which describe *The Four Elements.*

THE FOUR ELEMENTS

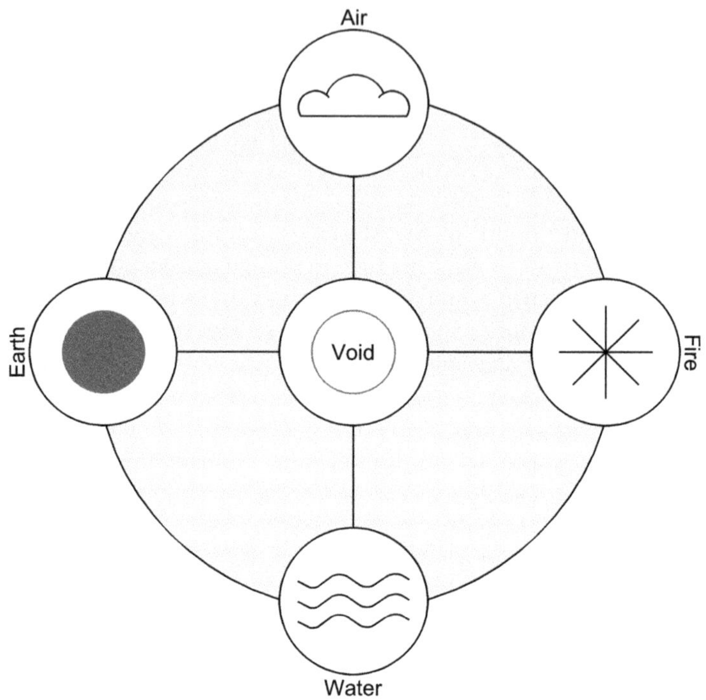

Figure 3.1 The Four Elements Illustrated by Ed England.

In the order of Creation, Air, Fire, Water, and Earth are the four elements. The fifth, or center of this wheel is the Void from and through which all elements were birthed.

In the diagram above, you will see the sigil which represents each of these elements. A sigil is a universally understood symbol and contains many levels of meaning that "unlock" our subconscious mind's interconnections to all forms of all things.

Notice where each of these elements are placed on the wheel. Their placement gives another layer of meaning to each of the four directions.

The South sings of the fluidity of WATER.
The West sings of the stability and endurance of the EARTH.
The North sings of the flexibility of the wind or of AIR.
The East sings of the expansion of FIRE.
The Center sings of the Black Hole, the Womb or the VOID.

THE ASPECTS OF BEING HUMAN

Within our make-up as human beings we can identify aspects of ourselves that are direct reflections of external aspects of nature. Contemplate the following:

The South is the EMOTIONAL aspect.
The heart reflects the song of the Water and the Moon.
In this way, we give with beauty.

The West is the PHYSICAL aspect.
The body reflects the song of the Earth, both element and planet.
In this way, we hold and transform with strength.

The North is the MENTAL aspect.
The mind reflects the song of the Wind or Air and the Stars.
In this way, we receive with clarity.

The East is the SPIRITUAL aspect.
The spirit reflects the song of the Fire and the Sun. In this way, we determine with responsibility.

The Center is the SEXUAL aspect.
The soul reflects the song of the Void and the Black Hole.
In this way, we catalyze with individuality.

THE GIFTS OF BEING HUMAN

When we accept these reflections and apply our free will choice to determine that our way is the Way of the Rainbow, we will sing the following song.

We will GIVE WITH TENDERNESS
by gathering together in our heart space.

We will HOLD WITH INTIMACY
by caring for one another's physical spaces.

We will RECEIVE WITH CARING
by teaching one another respect, honor and dignity.

We will DETERMINE WITH PASSION AND LUST
by sharing with one another our spiritual visions.

We will have OPEN HEART TO HEART COMMUNICATION
when we are intimate with one another.

The preceding quotation from Harley SwiftDeer Reagan's book *Shamanic Wheels and Keys*—The Four Elements, The Aspects of Being Human, The Gifts of Being Human–provide the cornerstone for the psychological foundations of the present book.

I invite the reader to become familiar with the quotation before reading my psychological understanding and interpretation of the quotation on the following pages.

With these very words, SwiftDeer introduced the Medicine Wheel to the wider world in the first edition of his book Shamanic Wheels and Keys in 1980. My heart is touched by the humanity of SwiftDeer's portrayal of *The Four Elements*, a soul in harmony with their community, the natural world, and the universe.

SwiftDeer's Sexual Aspect

SwiftDeer touches lightly on the masculine and feminine expressions of the Sexual aspect, discussed in detail in later paragraphs, the force and directionality of the masculine, the receptiveness and intimacy of the feminine.

He writes, 'we catalyze with individuality'. Catalysis means 'change caused by an agent which itself remains unchanged'.[2] So, I read 'we catalyze with individuality' as a reference to the force and directionality of the masculine expression of Sexuality.

When he writes, 'We will have open heart to heart communication when we are intimate with one another', I read this as a reference to the receptiveness and intimacy of the feminine expression of Sexuality.

The Dynamic Portrayal of Soul (See Figure below)

Feelings, Body, Mind, and Spirit in Metaphor

The elements of being—Feelings, Body, Mind, and Spirit—are represented metaphorically by the elements of water, earth, air, and fire, respectively.

Feelings flow like water. When we feel, we give something of ourselves. Intuition is similar to feelings, a sense of knowing something without knowing how.

Body has the strength and endurance to contain us and is the medium of expression for our feelings; we may weep when we are grieving, go red with rage, or smile when we are happy. The body includes our five senses and visceral senses. Intuition is experienced as a visceral sense, sometimes referred to as a 'gut feeling'.

Mind is as free as air to receive intelligence from our feelings, intuition, body, and environment, with the clarity to analyse this knowledge, to reflect upon it, and to formulate options.

Spirit is a transforming fire, using the knowledge our mind has received and formulated to make life choices, great and small, which determine our way in the world and our relationship with the world, the personality we present. Spirit has an expanding capacity to be self-reflective, make choices, exercise will, create change, and be self-determined.

Sexuality

The Dynamic Portrayal of Soul has Womb or Void, the Sexual Aspect, as the central point within a human being.

Sexuality is the central point to which everything is related and which is the source of energy infusing the whole being, feelings, body, mind, and spirit.

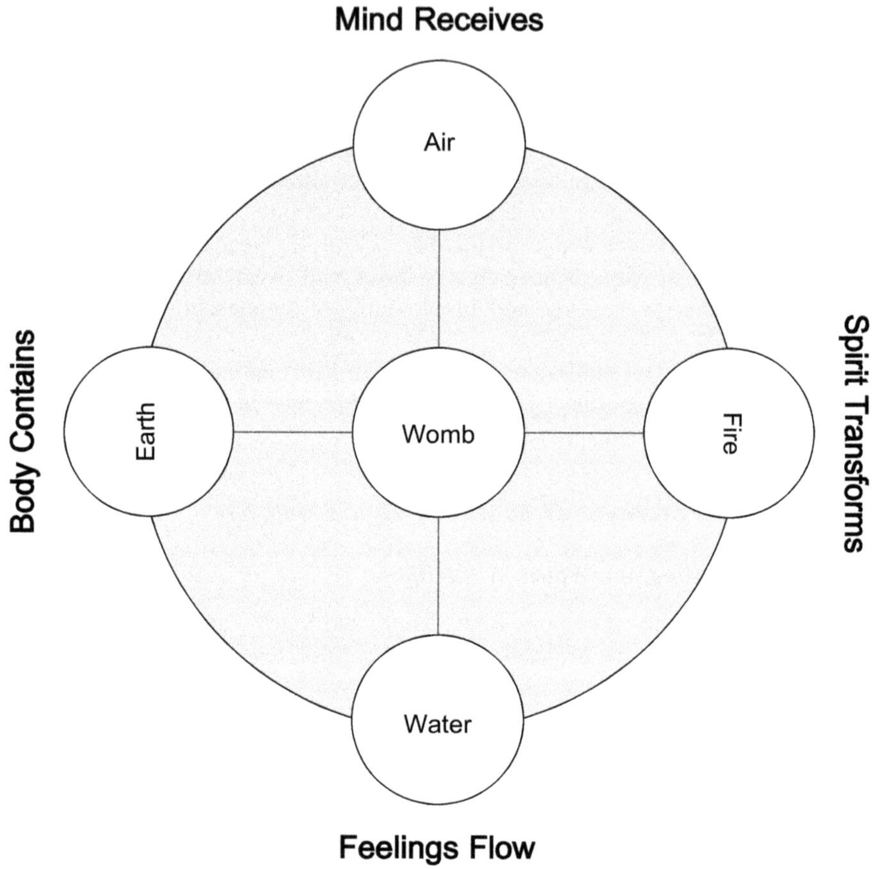

Figure 3.2 The Dynamic Portrayal of Soul Illustrated by Ed England.

Evolution of Sexuality: Energy for Life

At the centre of the Medicine Wheel is Sexuality. Sexuality originated with the evolution of the first self-reproducing organism 3.5 billion years ago, the common ancestor from which all life on Earth has descended. Sexuality is the life-force that has created and sustains every species of life on the planet, each with its own system of sexual reproduction.

Sexuality is the life-force that supplies energy for life, that vitality differentiating a living being from a lifeless corpse. We experience life-force simply by knowing we are alive.

The metaphor for Sexuality is an inviting void, a fertile womb; Sexuality is the vital energy that seemingly can form something wonderful out of nothing: a fertilised egg, a pollinated seed, an inspired thought.

Sexuality is "the force that through the green fuse drives the flower" (Dylan Thomas, 1952, p. 18). By photosynthesis, the flower converts electromagnetic light energy into chemical energy which, when combined with carbon dioxide and water, creates the carbohydrate molecules used to form the vegetative parts of the flower, petals and sepals, enclosing the sexual organs, carpels and stamens, that effect reproduction. Sexuality is the force and directionality driving the flower's reproduction. Indeed, *Sexuality is the force and directionality driving the reproduction of all plants and animals and the thread running throughout their evolution.*

To energise our body's cells we eat plants and inhale oxygen, the products and by-products of photosynthesis. So, the sun is our ultimate source of energy, energy moving into a myriad structures to synthesise and sustain our living being. Thus, *Sexuality is the life-force, energy for life, real energy, infusing our whole being*: the complex functioning of our body; the physiological processes that give us the experiences of feeling; and the brain functions that give us the experience of thinking.

Sexuality: Masculine Energy

The force and directionality of Sexuality, the masculine dimension, are active throughout life, engendering psychospiritual growth in the individual, and becomes most evident at a time of Soul Crisis. James Hillman offers a graphic description of Soul Crisis:

> Pathology is the place that keeps the person in the soul, that torment, that twist that you can't simply be naïve, you can't simply go along in a natural way, that there's something broken, twisted, hurting, that forces constant reflection. There's a work going on all the time, a fire burning, something elemental happening ... the soul's way of working on itself, the pathology necessary to that working of imagination.
>
> (Hillman, 1983, p. 23)

SOULMAKING: EXPANDING OF SPIRIT, DEEPENING OF SOUL

Soul is the experience of being alive, and Soul Crisis is a hiatus in that experience. The root of such 'pathology' is the force and directionality of Sexuality; keeping the person in the Soul serves to bring about transformation, a successful outcome being an expansion of Spirit and a deepening of the experience of being alive, a deepening of Soul.

The Soul Crisis is an agonising dialogue between Sexuality and Spirit. Sexuality is the force and directionality driving change, forcing reflection. Yet, change needs an act of determination and will by Spirit, the transforming fire, though this is not a foregone conclusion. We can distract ourselves, maybe through a recurring cycle of sexual relationships or by resorting to a pharmaceutical way of numbing ourselves from those disturbing feelings.

James Hillman's quotation serves to illustrate the dynamics of Soul Crisis, how disturbing Feelings (South on the Portrayal) are invoked to be expressed and contained in the Body (West), forcing reflection (North) and necessitating the working of imagination and will by Spirit (East). Pathology here is dis-ease, not disease, a normal functioning of *The Dynamic Portrayal of Soul* in a time of Soul Crisis. The Wheel goes around as we grow in Spirit, and as we grow in Spirit we deepen Soul. There's a work going on all the time, though rarely so dramatic as a Soul Crisis. The dialogue between Sexuality and Spirit goes on throughout life. We may receive promptings, experienced as a call or a sense of vocation or a sudden insight. Here is my personal testimony to the interplay between Sexuality and Spirit:

> Some years ago, I was feeling increasingly discontented with my work in IT, when a friend whom I had not seen for some time asked me, "What do you really want to do?" I replied without hesitation, and completely out of the blue, out of nowhere, "I want to be a psychologist," which surprised us both. "Well, that's interesting," she said, "Because I'm doing this course in Psychosynthesis." It was the first time I had heard the word. This brief exchange changed the direction of my life.

Change needs an act of determination and will by Spirit. This influences how we Feel about ourselves. Which influences how our Feelings are expressed in our Body and maybe our attitude to our Body. Changes in Feelings and Body influence the understanding our Mind has of ourselves. And so back to Spirit, the Wheel goes around, an expanding of Spirit, a deepening of Soul.

This is Soulmaking, discussed further in the *Journey of Soulmaking.*

Sexuality: Feminine Energy

The receptiveness and intimacy of sexuality, the feminine dimension, is about two-ness in relationship, intercourse, attachment, and nurture.

Receptiveness and intimacy in an encounter between two people: when we are intimate with one another, we have an open heart-to-heart connection, and we have intercourse. 'Intercourse' is from Latin *inter* 'between' plus *currere* 'to run'; intercourse is whatever runs or passes between people in their relationship; be it social contact, friendship, spiritual connection, or sexual union; in their encounter, the space between people is the fertile ground, the womb which sexual energy fills with life.

Receptiveness and intimacy in whatever runs or passes between mother and child: the mother nourishing the baby within her own body; the newborn seeking and attaching to mother's breast; the mother's loving gaze conveying her love to the infant self and receiving their love in response; and the attachment that an infant forms with mother.

Receptiveness and intimacy in our encounter with the natural world: in her Inkling *Bluebell Blessing*, psychotherapist and author Susan Holliday gives us an inkling of such an emotive encounter, "The wood lies unclad, like a baby. Naked as a nymph. In the presence of this undress I feel suddenly burdened with protective layers. Not only from the coat I wear, with its seal of water-proofing, but also from all the calcified layers of attitude and belief that have built up in me over sixty years of living in a world that has always felt too fast, too coarse and too concrete."

Receptiveness and intimacy in whatever runs or passes between therapist and client: The therapist affords their client 'unconditional positive regard'. The client comes to have a deep regard for their therapist, to trust them, and to share with them what they share with no other person.

The therapist expresses masculine energy in the way they are insightful and incisive, and feminine energy in the way they hold, mirror, love, and care for the client.

Sexuality: Feminine and Masculine Energy

Both receptive feminine energy and penetrating masculine energy are necessary for fertility, with procreation being both an example of and a metaphor for creative connection. The two-ness of intimate creative encounter transforms the void, the space between people, into a fertile womb to be impregnated by mutual penetration and reception, of inspired expression and reflective response.

Soulmaking: Expanding of Spirit, Deepening of Soul

Intimate creative encounter affects every part of our being, arousing Feeling, exciting Body, stimulating Mind, prompting Spirit to make a life choice, to embrace the two-ness of two. Feminine sexual energy is invigorating, breathtaking, and exhilarating, yielding an expansion of Spirit and a deepening of Soul.

Spirit

Spirit is a transforming fire. Spirit has an expanding capacity to be self-reflective, make choices, exercise will, create change, and be self-determined. It does so with the influence of Sexuality. The force and directionality of masculine sexual energy guides psychospiritual growth. The receptiveness and intimacy of feminine sexual energy encourages the two-ness of two in relationship, intercourse, attachment, and nurture. The guidance and encouragement of Sexuality yields an expansion of Spirit and a deepening of Soul.

At the same time, there is balance between the guidance and encouragement of Sexuality and Spirit's free will: to be self-reflective, make choices, exercise will, create change, and be self-determined. There is an ongoing dialogue between Sexuality and Spirit.

In differing ways, masculine and feminine energies influence Spirit. Spirit is further influenced by childhood conditioning and trauma. From childhood into adulthood, a person may feel of low self-worth, maybe: feeling rejected or unwanted; feeling needy and dependent; feeling emotionally abandoned; feeling possessed; feeling ashamed and body dysmorphic from being sexually abused; and all else that curbs the growth of Spirit and wounds Soul. People often express what they feel about themselves in the form of a succinct but false 'core myth'—I'm not good enough; there's something wrong with me; I'm unloveable; ...—a core myth that is the root of the maintaining cycle familiar to therapists.

Furthermore, adult trauma—physical, sexual, and domestic abuse, coercive control, and gaslighting—has the effect of distorting Spirit and wounding Soul.

Soul

Soul Experience

Whilst Feelings, Body, Mind, and Spirit are elements of being, and Sexuality is the source of energy infusing the whole being, Soul is the total package, our present, whole, lived experience of being a Soul.

Soul is contained within a flexible membrane, our skin, and Soul is our lived experience of being held within this membrane. Soul comprises everything experienced within the membrane, Feelings, Body, Mind, Spirit, Sexuality: our feelings, intuitions, imagination, the five senses, visceral senses, spatial awareness and balance, physical pain or discomfort or vitality, promptings or calls or sense of vocation, a sudden insight, thoughts, determinations, and so on.

Soul's Inner Being

Soul, the total package, our lived experience of being a Soul. Yet there is more, our inner being, hidden from our experience, whilst revealing itself to us through intuition, insight, imagination, inspiration, and dreams, and thereby coming within our Soul Experience.

Soul Connection: The Two-ness of Two Souls

Soul Connection is the two-ness of two souls coming into relationship. SwiftDeer doesn't include Soul in *The Four Elements* explicitly, yet two-ness is implicit in the Sexual Aspect, Gifts of Being Human, "We will have open heart to heart communication when we are intimate with one another." As relational beings, when we connect with another, we share something of each other's energy, if only a trace of memory. I sometimes enjoy brief 'cameo conversations', like this one:

> It is the middle of the night at Gatwick airport. I am waiting hours for my flight to be called, along with a million others, a living nightmare. I squeeze into a seat in a balcony café, with a cup of coffee. The woman sitting next to me turns towards me, locks eyes with me, and says, "This is the seventh circle of hell." Eye to eye, a brief Soul Connection, being in hell together. It lives in my memory.

We can enjoy Soul Connection not only with people; we can also connect with the natural world. Psychotherapist and author Susan Holliday writes about moments of intimate Soul Connection with the natural world in her collection of prose poems 'Inklings'. In *The Dark River*, for example, she captures a moment of interconnection with the life energy of a waterfall.

I feel a Soul Connection with mature trees, particularly when they occupy sacred sites: the 1,700-year-old yew tree in Compton Dundon churchyard, with messages strung from its branches; an age-old yew tree in, unusually, a circular churchyard at Aldworth in Berkshire, surrounded by a circle of holly bushes, an ancient sacred site long before the church was built.

Connecting deeply with another person is the two-ness of two souls, an exchange of energy. Something of their Soul becomes part of my Soul, and mine of theirs. For each of us this is a Soul Experience. Sometimes a two-ness can be spontaneous, like when there is sustained eye contact, such as these two memories of the two-ness of two souls:

> At a summer festival, I have a long conversation with a trans-man, a mature soul. Some time later, I happen to attend a workshop where this man is also present. We are paired up for an exercise involving sustained eye contact, the effect of prolonged eye contact being for us to feel deep connection and affection, like gazing into the other's soul.
>
> At another dance camp, in the grounds of Braziers Park Community Residential College, our 5Rhythms dance session is joined by residents. 5Rhythms includes short periods of dancing in couples, with dancers often reluctant to make eye contact. I dance with a woman from the college. It's like we spontaneously trust each other and are willing to maintain eye contact as we dance. The rhythm of the music, our movement in the dance, our touch, our sustained eye contact, form a gestalt, a five minute love affair. Then we part, as 5Rhythms moves on, never to meet again, yet in my case at least, always to remember our five minute love affair.

In a longer relationship, be it a friendship or a sexual union, the exchange of energy can include feelings of commitment, loyalty, trust, a sense of alignment, and a feeling of love:

> I spend a chaste weekend with a friend, unspokenly discovering we love each other. She and I enjoy simple pleasures, buying fish straight from the sea, cooking and eating the fish, drinking beer in a cosy bar, walking the promenade, attending a reading of poetry. An air of enchantment blows through all we take pleasure in. The rapture, such energy, is alive in my memory.

Two people can experience a profound level of Soul Connection when there is mutual trust, alignment, openness, and perhaps most of all authenticity: a deeply shared spiritual encounter; ineffable yet natural; rapturous yet grounded; expansive yet contained. This feminine dimension of Sexuality present in their lives is a call to Spirit, inviting them to determine the meaning of the Soul Connection, a creative call to give birth to some looked-for progeny.

The Journey of Soulmaking

The *Journey of Soulmaking* has its origins in *Principles of Transpersonal Psychology* (Laura Boggio Gilot, 1997) and *The Triphasic Model of Psychospiritual Enfoldment* (Joan Evans, 2021), taught in my psychotherapy training at the Institute of Psychosynthesis London.

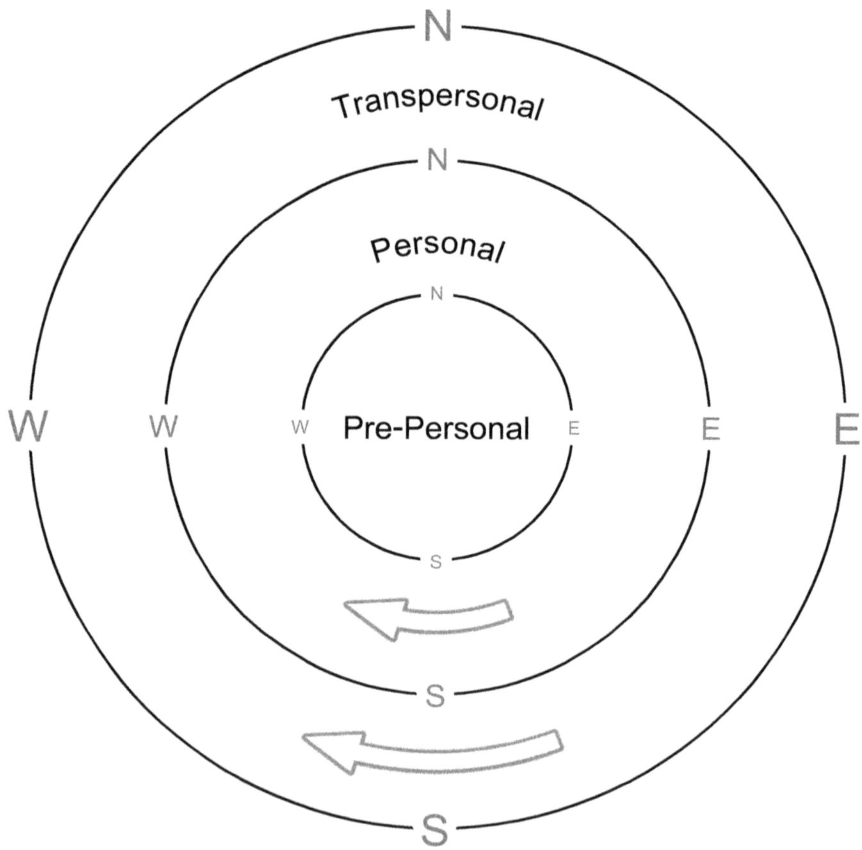

Figure 3.3 The Journey of Soulmaking Illustrated by Ed England.

The *Journey of Soulmaking* map (See above Figure) depicts the expansion of Consciousness and Will through three main phases of development:

Integration of a mature Ego, a Survival self, Conscious of having the Will to survive in the world;

Integration of a Personal self, Conscious of their capacity to be self-reflective, to recognise choice, and to exercise their Will to choose;

Integration of a Transpersonal self ('trans' from the Latin, meaning in this book both 'going beyond' and 'becoming'), increasingly Conscious of being part of the whole, of being Willing to be part of the whole, along with other people and other living things, to acknowledge and respect other people and other living things within the whole.

The core of the *Journey of Soulmaking* map can be summed up in two words: **differentiation** and **integration**. The process of **differentiation** and **integration** is fundamental to the *Journey of Soulmaking*.

Soulmaking

During the *Journey of Soulmaking*, the Wheel goes around, an expanding of Spirit, a deepening of Soul; this journey of soulmaking is the process of psychospiritual development happening throughout the three phases, which may be most evident to the therapist at a time of Soul Crisis, most likely towards the culmination of a phase—integrating a Survival self or integrating a Personal self—when a client may be in a state of torment and vulnerability.

The Process of Differentiation and Integration

The three phases are represented in the diagram opposite as three major rotations of the Medicine Wheel: Pre-personal, Personal, and Transpersonal. With each rotation of the Medicine Wheel there is an expanding of Spirit, a deepening of Soul.

The core of the *Journey of Soulmaking* can be summed up in two words: **differentiation** and **integration**.

The metaphor for each rotation is birth. In its beginning, an infant is fused with the mother, undifferentiated, having no sense of identity. Contingent upon the mother's ability to mirror the infant as he or she is reflected in mother's face,[3] fusion gives way to a symbiotic stage, where the child's identity is found in the relationship with mother, a gradual process of differentiation culminating in the integration of a sense of personal identity.

The Model in Mirrors

The *Journey of Soulmaking* is all about mirrors:

Pre-personal consciousness and will: Ego, or Survival self, is built by mirroring.

Personal consciousness and will: Personal self is attained by self-reflection.
Transpersonal consciousness and will: Self is realised by the individual seeing through the self-reflective mirror to the universal.

Pre-personal Consciousness and Will, and Ego Development

Ego/Survival Self is Built by Mirroring

Whenever a mother looks into her baby's eyes, she is mirroring her child. Through the quality of mirroring, the child comes to know themselves.

Children are impressionable and throughout childhood assimilate the 'way of being' of parents, family, and society in which they are growing up, its values, beliefs, attitudes, and aspirations. Then again, a family's 'way of being' is not always child friendly. The mother, father, and caregiver may offer an inauthentic mirror. Ill-treatment and neglect become part of what is assimilated, leaving the person with false beliefs about themselves. You've heard it: I am not good enough; I am unloveable; I don't need anybody…

Becoming mature means **differentiation** from fusion with mother and **integration** of a mature ego, Conscious of having the Will to survive in the world, a Survival self. The Survival self has the level of Consciousness and Will with which we enter adulthood, though some people continue in the Pre-personal phase well into adulthood.

A mature ego is able to survive in the world by following the 'way of being' they know, the 'way of being' they have assimilated throughout childhood.[4]

Our Role as Therapist

Contingent upon their mother's[5] ability to mirror them as an infant, an adult client may still be stuck psychologically in a symbiotic relationship with 'mother', being dependent upon parents, partners, or friends. Our role as therapist, at the Pre-personal phase, is to be an *authentic mirror*, serving to counteract any inauthentic mirroring in childhood. In the presence of a therapist who is attentive and empathic towards them in the suffering that brought them into therapy, the client can come to see and know something of their true nature and to know they have the Will to survive in the world.

Personal Consciousness and Will, and The Development of Personal Self

Personal Self Is Attained by Self-reflection

Whilst a person has the Will to survive in the world, the Survival self still runs on rails, restricted to the tracks laid down in their assimilated 'way of being', with their system of values, beliefs, attitudes, aspirations, and their false beliefs about themselves. The Survival self is an egoic false self.

This is the state of fusion at the start of the second phase, an egoic false self stuck in the assimilated 'way of being' they acquired as they grew up.

The Personal phase involves **differentiation**, from fusion with the 'way of being' of the Survival self to the **integration** of the Personal self.

The process of **differentiation** is characterised by: increasing Consciousness; a capacity for self-reflection; and the Will to make life choices. The culmination of this phase is the **integration** of a Personal self, whose capacity for self-reflective thought enables them to recognise choice and to exercise their Will to choose.

The Personal self, as shown in the above diagram, transcends, contains, and moderates the Pre-personal self, retaining the ego's capacity and Will to survive in the world. The Personal self has an increasing capacity to question the Survival self's assimilated system of values, beliefs, attitudes, and aspirations, and to choose differently. One of the choices the Personal self can make, is to set aside false beliefs in favour of right beliefs: I am good enough; I am loveable; I need others to make my life complete…

Our Role as Therapist

Our role as therapist, at the Personal phase, whilst still providing an *authentic mirror*, is to be a *carer of Soul*, to support the client in broadening and deepening their Soul, their present, whole, lived experience of themselves, healing and expanding Soul as they grow in self-worth and self-esteem, self-awareness and self-will.

Transpersonal Consciousness and Will, and Self-Realisation

Self Is Realised by the Individual Seeing Through the Self-reflective Mirror to the Universal

Whilst the Personal self can make choices and exercise Will, they view the world from their subjective personal perspective. When we choose our opinion about something, arrived at through self-reflection, we can typically be self-assertive, pressing our opinion upon others. Self-reflection sometimes means a self-reflective mirror. This wilful self is an egotistical self, with an overwhelming sense of their own centrality. I remember wondering how people could go on existing outside of my presence. This is the state of fusion at the start of the third phase.

When I thought about the Transpersonal, I recalled from childhood being told, "Don't show off." What this does is to encourage false modesty. Actually, saying to oneself, I have reached the Transpersonal phase, can only be true when spoken with humility. Someone pointed out to me, the Transpersonal is not better than the Personal. The Personal is not better than the Pre-personal. These are just phases in a psychospiritual journey.

The Transpersonal phase involves **differentiation** from fusion with the egotistical Personal self. The *Journey of Soulmaking* is a lifelong Transpersonal journey towards Self-realisation; we spend the rest of our lives **Integrating** our sense of wholeness within ourselves, with others, and with the natural world.

The process of **differentiation** is characterised by: increasing Consciousness; a facility to see through the self-reflective mirror; and increasing knowledge of being Willing to be part of the whole, along with other people and other living things.

The Transpersonal self increasingly possesses: a sense of self; a sense of integrity; the reception, expression, and communication of emotions and feelings; the ability to regulate stress; empathy with others; compassion for others; a sense of humour; insight, intuition, and creativity.

Engaging with another at the Transpersonal phase means: expressing our point of view with integrity; being willing to listen and seek to understand another's point of view; recognising another's right to their point of view, without offering a counterargument, yet being willing to engage openly with them towards a synthesis of their differing points of view.

The Transpersonal self, as shown in the above diagram, transcends, contains, and moderates the Personal self, retaining the capacity of the Personal self to be self-reflective, to recognise choice, and to have the Will to make choices.

On the journey of becoming, I need to acknowledge and respect my integrity—as a unique, separate, and independent self within the whole—before I am equipped to acknowledge and respect another's integrity—as a unique, separate, and independent self within the whole—and by the same token to acknowledge and respect other living things within the whole. We are becoming free to relate to one another, to agree to work together, and to love each other and all living things, without ego projection or subjective personal assertion.

My Testimony: The Meaning of Life

It's my fifth year in secondary school. I make a list of the subjects I stand a chance of qualifying in, where my effort will be applied, which doesn't include geography. At the end of autumn term, my geography teacher Mr Warburton says to me in open class, "England, you're going to fail this examination if you're not careful." Just this! It awakens a new confidence in me. I pass in geography. At year end, my head teacher (aka Bachus) writes in red ink on my annual report, "It is a waste of time England going into the 6th Form." But, with the sustained confidence inspired in me by Mr Warburton, I do so anyway. Mr Warburton's gift is part of the social heritage, which, with my genetic and familial heritage, has served to shape the person I am. My maternal grandfather was an especial influence; he saw and heard me, and I have always seen him as my saviour.

My view of my life used to be just birth and everything in between until death. I now see this singular view as being, in its way, egotistical. My view of my life now, from a transpersonal viewpoint, is as part of a continuum, as a unique, separate, and independent life within the whole flow of human existence and beyond. Within this flow, as well as my genetic and familial heritage, I inherit from many who have been a significant influence, like Mr Warburton, and I am here to provide a genetic, familial, and social inheritance to those who follow after. The words of Dag Hammarskjöld (1963, p. 136) ring true for me, "Do not seek death. Death will find you. But seek the road which makes death a fulfilment." For me, this is the meaning of life.

Our Role as Therapist

Our role as therapist, whilst still being an *authentic mirror* and *carer of soul*, is to be a *gatekeeper*, one who opens gates along the client's path, being someone who has passed along a similar path; the *gatekeeper* supports the client to pass through the gate into a realisation of being part of the whole, along with other people and other living things.

The transpersonal is about relationship, with others and other living things, and as the therapy unfolds our role as therapist becomes *fellow traveller*, walking alongside the client, supporting one another through the relational hazards, snares, and pitfalls on the unending journey towards Self-realisation, the journey of soulmaking.

Psychotherapy with Soul

Finally, we need to further consider our role as therapist with the core psychology set out in this part of the section.

The *Journey of Soulmaking* is a practical dynamic model, and the growth of a person's Consciousness and Will—it needs to be emphasised—is not a sequential process; a person, for example, may be well advanced in seeing through to the universal and yet have unresolved issues at the Pre-personal phase. All the same, the model may provide a helpful indication of an individual's Centre of Gravity, the phase or rotation in which the client is predominantly located in their journey of life.

Tri-focal Vision

As therapist, we need to maintain 'tri-focal vision' throughout a client session, asking ourselves, which of the three phases is the client working in right now? This means our role as therapist is to be simultaneously an *authentic mirror*, a *carer of Soul*, a *gatekeeper*, and a *fellow traveller*. In this work, *The Journey of Soulmaking* is a practical guide to help us orient ourselves in our work.

Sexuality: Consciousness and Will

Sexuality is the dynamic central point within the psyche to which everything is related, the source of energy, the rotating engine driving the expansion of consciousness and will. Sexuality is an active force within the psyche that directs the development of both consciousness *and* will throughout the life of a person.

Sexuality directs development of consciousness and will, but human beings are not automata; they have free will; it is the person themself who, in consciousness, exercises will: the survival-self asserts the will to survive in the world; the Personal Self recognises choice and asserts the will to choose; and the Transpersonal Self asserts the will to be part of the whole, along with other people, other living things, and other lives past and future.

The nature of Sexuality, in its dual purpose of deepening and expanding of consciousness and of unfolding will, is to seek Self-realisation.

Songs of Being Human

SwiftDeer's description of *The Four Elements* refers to the songs of the four elements and the song of the womb or void. To complete *A Portrait of Soul*, I invite you to reflect on these five verses, a cryptic distillation of *The Dynamic Portrayal of Soul*. These verses express my sense of reverence for the aspects of being human: feelings, body, mind, spirit, and sexuality.

Feelings, Water: Song of the Water and the Moon

Shades of light and dark.
Circle dance of moon and tide.
Tears of pain and joy.

Body, Earth: Song of the Earth

Earth's a water pot.
Reservoir, river, or sea
Pouring on the earth.

Mind, Air: Song of the Wind or Air and Stars

Wind beneath its wings.
Intent on touching the stars,
Hawk's eyes scan the earth.

Spirit, Fire: Song of the Fire and the Sun

The soul lies in light.
The wind sows seeds of passion.
Enlightenment flowers.

Sexuality, Void: Song of the Void or Womb

Perpetual space,
Place of nurture, space to grow,
Life swells into being.

Notes

1 Deer Tribe Metis Medicine Society is a shamanic tradition inspiring spiritual evolution and dedicated to sharing Knowledge that Works which guides us into Healing, Growth and Transformation. Deer Tribe Metis Medicine Society has its Lodges throughout the world. https://dtmms.org/.
2 Online Etymology Dictionary.
3 Or father or main carer. Babies discern eye contact at two to five days, creating a sense of closeness and intimacy and serving to develop their social brain.
4 I wonder, when a person with a survival self meets someone they don't know, do they project onto them someone they do know to help them decide how safe they feel with them?.
5 Or main carer, sometimes father.

Bibliography

England, David (2017) *Soulfulness: The Marriage of Shamanic and Contemporary Psychology*, Routledge.
Evans, Joan (2021) The Triphasic Model of Psychospiritual Enfoldment. In Nocelli, Petra Guggisberg (Ed.), *Know, Love, Transform Yourself, Theory, techniques and new developments in Psychosynthesis* Vol. I, Psychosynthesis Books.
Gilot, Laura Boggio (1997) Principi di psicologia transpersonale [Principles of transpersonal psychology], Edizioni AIPT.
SwiftDeer Reagan, Harley (1980) *Shamanic Wheels and Keys*, Deer Tribe Metis Medicine Society.
Thomas, Dylan (1952) *The Poems of Dylan Thomas*, New Directions 2003.

Storytelling as a Healing Art

Storytelling as a Healing Art presents my perception of the relationship between storytelling and psychology, my appreciation of how stories have a healing power. I summarise with the maxim: *The story is the healer.*

Storytelling as a Healing Art then sets out the seven guiding precepts underpinning this maxim which have informed me in writing this book.

Soul and Soulmaking

I speak not about *having* a Soul but *being* a Soul; Soul as our present, whole, lived experience of being ourselves. As we develop and grow through life emotionally and psychologically, we deepen this experience of being who we are, we deepen Soul. Soulmaking (Hillman, 1989) is deepening our experience of being alive, and in the context of this section, Soulmaking through Story.

Soul and Imagination

In Soulmaking through Story, this is my first guiding precept:

The story is the healer; the story touches the Soul.

James Hillman makes the link between Soul and imagination, "soul is the imaginative possibility of our natures" (1989, p. 21), and he speaks of the capacity of the Soul to be moved (1975, p. 97).

One summer, my work in the healing area of the Oxford Dance Camp included telling earth tales to individuals and couples. I made it clear: I am not the healer, the story is the healer.

Sometimes, I would tell a story which touched the Soul, the listener felt moved by the story, and something moved within the listener's imagination; they would tell me later how the story went on working in them. A woman said to me, after listening to *Bee, Mantis, and Flower*,

"I heard it as a story about finding a place to rest after long labour, and *that* being the beginning of everything." The story is told. In a moment of imaginative possibility, something working in the imagination touches and moves the Soul, it

DOI: 10.4324/9781003712329-5

is "the beginning of everything". Soulmaking is what the healing art of storytelling is about.

The Sin Against the Imagination

In Soulmaking through Story, this is my second guiding precept:

We sin against the imagination when we ask a story for its meaning.

James Hillman (1975, p. 39) writes this, "We sin against the imagination when we ask an image for its meaning." We might pick apart the story of *Bee, Mantis, and Flower*, analyse it intellectually: what does Bee represent, what does Mantis represent, and how are we to interpret 'the Maker of Fire, the Keeper of the Dream'? If we pick apart the story, what are we left with? We take the life out of it. The story becomes a corpse dissected on the slab. We lose the Soul experience; we lose the imaginative possibility of the story moving us and working in our imagination.

A New Gestalt: A New Way of Experiencing Ourselves

In Soulmaking through Story, this is my third guiding precept:

Let the story tell the story.

The story enables the listener to generate a new way of experiencing themselves, which at the outset is unknown.

There's a splendid book called *The Springboard* by Stephen Denning (2000). It's a business book. In it Stephen describes how he discovered the power of storytelling to bring about organisational change and to communicate knowledge. Much of what he says is relevant to psychological change and the discovery of personal knowledge. He says,

> "When the story rings true, it enables the listeners to generate a new gestalt in their minds, which embraces the main point of the change." Or in my words, a new way of experiencing ourselves.
>
> "The immersion of the self in the events that constitute the story can have an impact. To follow a story as a listener is to participate in a conceptual journey, leading to a destination that at the outset is unknown to the listener." Or in my words, a new way of experiencing themselves, a new gestalt.

Reality and Imagination

In Soulmaking through Story, holding the thought of a reflective moment of imaginative possibility, this is my fourth guiding precept:

As everything begins in the imagination,
healing begins in the imagination.

James Hillman, as we have seen, makes the link between Soul and imagination, recognising, he says, all realities as first and foremost symbolic or metaphorical. Reality exists first in the imagination. Everything begins in the imagination.

> *I heard a story about Isambard Kingdom Brunel. Before he designed the Clifton suspension bridge, he had himself hauled across the Clifton gorge in a barrel. He experienced the gap for himself before applying himself to how it might be bridged. With this experience of the gorge, he was able to conceive the bridge in the imagination. So, what is more real, the external form of the bridge, or the concept upon which that form relies? Certainly, the concept has stood the test of time.*

Everything begins in the imagination, even the Clifton suspension bridge. In experiencing the gap, Brunel connected with the imaginative possibility of bridging it.

The imagination is inherent in our very experience of being human, our experience of Soul. Being so intimately familiar, the imagination is easily taken for granted, yet it is a strange and mysterious territory.

The imagination can disturb our dreams and fuel our anxieties. I experience this in myself. I see it in my psychotherapy clients all the time.

On the other hand, the imagination can captivate and enthral us and engender those sublime moments of creative insight, moments of grace.

We cannot control the imagination; it seems to have a mind of its own, a life of its own. Yet we can cooperate with it, set it on a path, follow its stream of images as they unfold, and have some choice over the path to follow through its labyrinth.

This is the sort of imaginative work therapists do with their clients, and sometimes it feels right simply to tell a story. Because, in its strange and mysterious way, the imagination can heal our brokenness by creating a new gestalt, a new way of experiencing ourselves.

To be healed, we need to imagine ourselves healed; therapists ask their clients this type of question, "What would it be like for you if…" A story can serve this act of imagination, and this is Soulmaking.

Stories State Existential Dilemmas

In Soulmaking through Story, this is my fifth guiding precept:

A story can state an existential dilemma briefly and pointedly,
in a way which resonates with the client's own inner conflicts,
so they can imagine themselves healed and being whole.

When thinking about the relationship between therapy and storytelling, Bruno Bettelheim's book *The Uses of Enchantment* (1991) is a helpful text.

> Bettelheim sees the 'fairy tale' as having been moulded through many generations to reflect a desirable solution to a universal human problem. So, the fairy tale becomes the purveyor of deep insights which are revealed simply and directly.
>
> He says, fairy tales speak to us in the language of symbols representing unconscious content. Their appeal is simultaneously to our conscious and unconscious mind.

> He explains how it is characteristic of fairy tales to state an existential dilemma briefly and pointedly, so that the hearer can come to grips with the problem in its most essential form.

So, fairy stories often concern a quite specific problem which the hero or heroine faces in their life. For example, Hansel and Gretel face the problem of abandonment, Snow White faces the experience of a jealous mother, and Ashputtel suffers neglect and exploitation.

In his elegant and humane book *Character Styles,* Stephen Johnson (1994) puts forward a theory of character formation in terms of the life issues which a child may face during their childhood, such as neglect, emotional abandonment, or exploitation by parents. (See Table below)

Johnson uses descriptive and imaginative names for those suffering from corresponding life issues: the schizoid character style he calls the Hated Child, the oral character style he calls the Abandoned Child, and so on, imaginative names.

I have brought together Johnson's approach and the idea of stories addressing existential problems; here are examples of stories, some included in this collection, which reflect life issues faced by clients.

A character style is a survival self, an adaptive personality with which the child identifies for their survival. Hearing the story, the client can identify with the hero or heroine who shares their existential dilemma. The story, with its transformative outcome, provides a different perspective, apprehended emotionally and spiritually, a new gestalt.

The Hansel & Gretel story, for example, accurately reflects the dilemma of the Abandoned Child:

> The Abandoned Child, having been emotionally abandoned repeatedly, is reluctant to trust anybody—including their therapist. The story is characterised by the total absence of a good mother in any form whatsoever, no fairy godmother, no wishing tree growing on the good mother's grave. Instead, when the children trust the nice old woman in the woods, Hansel says, this must be heaven, but she turns out to be a predatory witch. This is the repeated experience of an abandoned child.

Table 4.1 Character Styles and Stories

Character Style	*Existential Issue*	*Imaginative Name*	*Story*
Schizoid	Fear	Hated Child	*The Juniper Tree*
Oral	Abandonment	Abandoned Child	*Hansel & Gretel*
Narcissistic	Self-esteem	Used Child	*The Brave Little Tailor*
Borderline/dependent	Self-boundaries	Owned Child	*The Feeling In Her Bones*
Masochistic	Freedom	Defeated Child	*Wild Swans*
Oedipal	Love/sex	Exploited child	*Ashputtle*

> As with many abandoned children, the story is about addiction, and specifically about food. The story is set in a time of famine. The children fall upon the gingerbread house with bulimic glee. Gretel puts aside her own bodily needs, and lives on crayfish shells, whilst she fattens up Hansel for the oven, anorexic and bulimic. At a turn of the spiral, the children fall upon the witch's jewels with the same bulimic glee as they had the gingerbread house. In a transformative outcome, Gretel attains discretion, restraint, and will, letting the white bird carry them home across a lake one at a time.

Bettelheim says: The fairy tale is therapeutic because the listener finds their *own* solutions, through contemplating what the story seems to imply about them and their inner conflicts at this moment in their life.

In other words, the story resonates with the listener's Soul, and in this is its healing power. The story helps the listener imagine themselves healed, imagine themselves being whole.

The Resonance of a Story

In Soulmaking through Story, a *reflective* moment of imaginative possibility, this is my sixth guiding precept:

The right story holds up a mirror to the client's existential experience, and it is this which brings healing and transformation.

Metaphorically, a psychotherapist holds the space and mirrors the client. This story of an owned child recounts how telling a story can be a mirror for a client.

An Owned Child

One day, let's call her Dolores,[1] walks into a library and sees a notice titled 'Psychotherapy'. She says to herself,

"Psychotherapy, that's what my husband says I need." Later that day, she phones me for an appointment. Dolores enters psychotherapy believing that her husband owns her, because he tells her so, and that her father owned her before that and passed her on to him at their marriage. She is an Owned Child.

During two years of work in psychotherapy, Dolores' sense of autonomy and identity greatly increases. Nevertheless, she speaks about her body being cut off from the neck, and how she ignores it, neither adorns it nor even looks at it. She sums up her body image in a single word, 'withered'.

On the brink of adolescence, wanting to look attractive, Dolores had saved up for a fashionable short black dress with a white collar. When her father saw her wearing it for the first time, he said he was disgusted, and if she wore such a dress she would be ogled at. In that fragile moment of opening, when she needed her father to reflect her attractiveness, to enjoy her loveliness, to prize her, and to be a safe place for her to discover her sexuality, he failed her. He shattered her moment of opening, turning it into an experience for her of prurience and 'cringing shame'. He wounded her, and while telling the story she makes a stabbing movement towards her heart.

Dolores' story seems to me to resonate with the story *The Feeling In Her Bones*—in the *Tales of Soul Room*—so I tell her the story.

A Woman Who Is Not Owned

Dolores listens intently to the story, and in doing so she makes it her own. She empathises with the daughter 'tossed away' by her father. She connects with her own sense of her 'withered and skeletal body'. She physically cringes at the crabs eating the woman's flesh, saying,

"I know the feeling of being nibbled away at."

Dolores realises that being tossed away by her father was not only a single devastating incident but a process throughout her childhood; he never supported or acknowledged her, never attended her school functions, and never prized her. As I listen to her story, she leans towards me and says,

"I know I am growing flesh."

Soon after, she speaks of her newly decorated shower room's 'virginal' quality. I invite her to describe the Virgin.

"She is whole," she says, "She is warm, soft, tender, confident, with a core of wisdom and knowledge". My mirroring of these 'feminine qualities' invokes a conflict within her body, between the Complete Virgin and the Spoilt Virgin, 'wizened, ugly and black', as if these parts are struggling to possess and own her body. As we dialogue between the Complete Virgin and the Spoilt Virgin, I begin to say something,

"The Virgin is ...", without knowing how I shall finish the sentence, until the needful words surface,

"The Virgin is a woman who is not owned."

We have a spontaneous, deeply felt, shared moment of clarity and recognition.

Soon after, Dolores has the most beautiful dream of forget-me-nots unfurling from her body in waves: forget-me-not, forget-me-not.

The Story As Container

In Soulmaking through Story, this is my seventh guiding precept:

The story is the healer
and serves as a container for each hearer's Soul energy.

As a therapeutic vehicle, the story of *Vasilisa and Baba Yaga*—in the *Tales of Soul Room*—is the most powerful story I know. I sometimes tell the story as a form of guided meditation. I invite the group to make themselves comfortable, close their eyes, and allow themselves to watch the story unfold, noticing which part of the story has the strongest resonance for them. One woman was reluctant to attend, but later, when she shared her experience of the meditation, she said, triumphantly,

"I came home with the fire."

She later told me, the Vasilisa meditation had been a turning point in her life.

As a storyteller, it is important for me to remember this, remember to hold the story as a container, and to hold my own interpretation of the story lightly, because I don't know what the listeners need to take from the container, and I don't know what may touch the Soul.

Tess of the D'Urbervilles

The symbolic language of images and metaphors, when employed therapeutically, has the capacity to bring healing. The healing process involves containing the powerful and difficult energies in the psyche, releasing and transforming them, and bringing meaning and understanding to the client.

Here is another example of the story as a container for Soul energy:

> One of my psychotherapy clients finds it too difficult, too frightening, to speak directly of the sexual violation which she has suffered. So, we talk instead about Thomas Hardy's *Tess of the d'Urbervilles: A Pure Woman* (1891): Tess's exploitive parents; her violation by a man she trusted; her life experience of repeated exploitation, rejection, and violation; how she embraces guilt, shame, degradation, and finally the abject abandonment of her values and self-worth; then, the restoring of her innocence—represented by her younger sister—and the redeeming of a healthy relationship with the masculine.

Using this story as a container enabled the client to release the energies of her violation with safety and to understand and come to terms with her own life's story.

Therapeutic Storywriting: Writing One's Own Story

So far, the discussion has been about the healing art of telling stories. A section on storytelling as a healing art would be incomplete, however, without considering the healing power of writing one's own fairy story.

Dr Trisha Waters,[2] the author of *Therapeutic Storywriting* (2004), works therapeutically with children, encouraging them to write stories "within the protected world of the imaginary". She says,

> "By playing with different characters, scenes, and plots of which they are the creators, storywriting seems to provide a way for the child to explore who they are and what they feel within the protected world of the imaginary, providing the opportunity to express their internal world through story metaphor."

The following telling comment by a 10-year-old child illustrates the capacity of the child's own written story to contain difficult energies:

> "It's for people who may have had a few problems and need someone to talk to. You can write stories and talk about problems but don't have to say it's you."

This is how a child's storywriting provides containment: you can talk about problems but don't have to say it is you.

So, using Trisha's words, "the symbolic language of story, of monsters and mythical creatures, of heroes and heroines, of terrifying obstacles overcome, can convey meaning more powerfully to a child than the best thought-out rational arguments."

Trisha Waters has kindly given me permission to reproduce the following extract from her book *Therapeutic Storywriting* (pp. 11–12).[3] This illustrates the therapeutic power of storywriting, enabling a child, Anya, to explore who she is and what she feels within the protected world of the imaginary, providing for her an opportunity to express her internal world through story metaphor.

Anya's Story, "We've Been Eaten"

"Anya was a Year 6 girl who had become a selective mute in the classroom following traumatic events at home, where she now lived with just her mother and sister. Her class teacher said she would not speak to her 'even to say yes or no' and mostly would just sit and not attempt her work at all. The most response she would give was a shrug of the shoulders. At times she would become completely stubborn and have uncontrollable temper tantrums which led to the teacher having to remove the rest of the children from the classroom on a couple of occasions. Anya had witnessed a serious traumatic incident at home a few years earlier and also had tantrums at home. She had been referred to a therapist out of school but would not speak during these sessions and they were discontinued after a few visits.

In the first group session Anya attended she did not speak, and when I asked her to get her writing equipment, she didn't move. I gently asked her again if she could get these, whereupon she became tearful. I thought she might be unwell and took her to the medical room. However, 10 minutes later the secretary came in to tell me that she was having a huge tantrum—hysterically screaming and kicking the wall. The second week Anya arrived but would not sit down with the rest of the group. When I approached her to quietly ask if she was all right, she physically withdrew and hunched up her shoulders. Again she had tears in her eyes and looked frightened. I told her that it was OK for her to stand there and that we would just get on with the lesson. I pointed out that there was a seat next to me when she was ready to join us. I was impressed at the ability of the other group members to accept this and continue the group work without comment.

The next week, Anya came in and sat next to me. The group were writing their own stories based on a well-known fairytale. While Anya again did no writing, she did appear to be listening to the stories that were shared. Another session went by when Anya again just came in and silently sat next to me. However, the next week she came in, picked up her pen and wrote the following story based on the story of the Three Bears:

We've Been Eaten

Hello I am Ginger bread 1. We were just asleep on the table after eating dinner. We could not go to bed. We were too tired even to walk upstairs.

Suddenly a girl jumped in through our window which made me wake up but I lay still just in case. She fell asleep in baby bread's bed, woke up and tried out my bed and ginger bread 2's bed. Then she sat on baby bread's chair and broke it. After that she rejected my chair and ginger bread two's chair. Then she started nibbling baby breads toes and up and up and up. So now baby bread was eaten. Then she ate gingerbread two—and now she is eating me. She is eating my little toes and now is up to my knees. Being eaten, as you know, is very painful. You just wish they would hurry up and eat you all up. I'm afraid I can not speak anymore because I'm very nearly eaten.

[The following week] Anya brought in the picture [of her story] and, speaking to me for the first time in four weeks, told me in a whisper that she had done it on her computer at home.

Over the following six months Anya continued to engage with writing and gradually began to speak in school. Her tantrums became less frequent."

This remarkable story *We've Been Eaten* illustrates, through writing stories as well as telling them, all of the seven precepts of storytelling as a healing art discussed in this paper.

Notes

1 A typical client.
2 Director, Centre for Therapeutic Storywriting, TherapeuticStorywriting.co.uk.
3 Dr Trisha Waters' copyright of the quoted text is hereby acknowledged.

Bibliography

Bettelheim, Bruno (1989) *The Uses of Enchantment*, Vintage.

Denning, Stephen (2000) *The Springboard: How Storytelling Ignites Action in Knowledge-Era Organizations*, Routledge.

Hardy, Thomas (1891) *Tess of the d'Urbervilles: A Pure Woman*, Penguin Classics (published 2003).

Hillman, James (1975) *Re-visioning Psychology*, Harper Perennial.

Hillman, James (1989) *The Essential James Hillman: A Blue Fire*, Routledge.

Johnson, Stephen (1994) *Character Styles*, W. W. Norton.

Waters, Trisha (2004) *Therapeutic Storywriting: A Practical Guide to Developing Emotional Literacy in Primary Schools*, David Fulton. www.TherapeuticStorywriting.co.uk

Part II

Rooms

Storytelling from a Psychotherapy Perspective: Bawdy and Beastly Tales is a browsing book. You are invited to visit the *Catalogue of Stories in the Collection* and to choose a Room to browse in or a story to peruse. There is a lot to choose from, 6 rooms and 50 stories: Bawdy Tales Room, Beastly Tales Room, Transpersonal Tales Room, Tales of Soul Room, Original Stories Room, Storytelling with Children Room.

Each story is self contained, including, with some variations: an abstract, my preamble, a synopsis of the story, the story itself, my sources, i.e. where I found the story to retell in my own words, and accompanying psychological reflections: My Psychological Reflections, Egalitarian Reflections, and suggestions as to Your Psychological Reflections.

As with a painting in an exhibition, you are offered—in the story and its reflections—an immersive imaginative and emotional experience, the feelings and visceral senses, thoughts, images, and intuitions which the story evokes, from which you can take what you need from the story and grasp the psychological meaning the story has for you.

Note, A Plague on Plagiarism*: From time to time, when I read a traditional tale or hear it told, the tale will grab me, like it demands to be told, so I take the plot and retell the tale in my own words. This is the living tradition of storytelling. All the traditional tales appearing in this book were written by me for the purpose of my storytelling performances, and are in my own words. The 'Sources' paragraph for each story records where I came across the story and where you can find other versions of the story.*

DOI: 10.4324/9781003712329-6

Bawdy Tales Room

On rare occasions, I have been allowed the ultimate privilege that a man can be afforded, to sit in on women's talk, so fast and fluid, so effortlessly comic, so sublimely bawdy. I hope these tales exude something of the same spirit. To my mind and heart, the traditional tales in this section are an acknowledgement of the skilful will, moral strength, incisive wit, and acute inner wisdom possessed by women and embodied in women's sexuality.

> *A woman in a garden gives an apple to a man. Blow away the moralistic misogyny clouding this image for millennia. A woman in a garden gives an apple to a man, an image of unashamed, enchanting sexuality, and the true creation myth is revealed.*
>
> *The women in this Room speak for themselves. These tales recognise the skilful will, moral strength, incisive wit, and acute inner wisdom possessed by women and embodied in women's sexuality.*

Psychological and Egalitarian Reflection

The woman in the therapy room—yours or mine—however clouded by ill-treatment and neglect, needs to be *seen* by the therapist, *seen* as the woman she can be, an unashamedly, enchantingly sexual woman, if she is to see herself and own the qualities she possesses. Psychotherapy is an act of imagination.

DOI: 10.4324/9781003712329-7

The Crane's Leg

I have told 'The Crane's Leg' several times as part of bawdy tales performances, but as I was trying to put together the 'Bawdy Tales Room', I struggled with this story; it just didn't seem to work. Then, my son Ed, who has edited all my published books, made the enlightened suggestion that it would work better in the first person. 'The Crane's Leg' is her story.

Let the story tell the story.
The story enables the listener to generate a new way of experiencing themselves, which at the outset is unknown.

Synopsis

A Tuscan noble's hawks bring down a plump crane, which he sends to his cook to have ready for the evening's feast. As the cook is roasting the bird and preparing it for the table, its aromas, wafting through the kitchens, catch the nose of the pastry cook, who entices the cook into sharing a thigh with her in return for a taste of her figgy pudding. The Tuscan noble is displeased to discover, when carving the crane at table, that it has only one leg. Called to account to his master for the missing leg, the cook insists that a crane only has one leg. Early the following morning, by the river, where noble, cook, and cranes gather, the Tuscan noble plans revenge and humiliation. Then comes the life-changing denouement.

The Story

Currado owns a grand Tuscan mansion on the banks of the River Arno. His love of hawks and horses is exceeded only by his fame for the splendour of his lavish feasts. Of course, he employs the greatest chef in all the land, Giovanni. I've watched Giovanni rise; I've watched others rise too, but I've chosen him, as we women do; he's the one for me.

On the hunting field today, Currado's falcons bring down a plump crane, known for having the tastiest meat of all wild game. He has it delivered to Giovanni with instructions to roast it with the greatest delicacy. Roasted to perfection, tender and juicy, its aromas drift through the kitchens. Giovanni sets the crane to stand while he prepares truffle sauce and tender asparagus, before dressing the dish for the table.

I'm Brunette, a pastry cook, famous for my figgy pudding, so soft and moist and sweet, the perfect dessert to complement the bird. Drawn by the delicate aromas of roasted crane, I enter Giovanni's kitchen and draw close to him. This is my chance.

"Mm!" I say, brushing closer to Giovanni, "if this bird tastes as toothsome as its aroma, let's share a thigh together."

"Absolutely not," replies a scandalised Giovanni, "this dish is for Currado's table."

"Come on, Giovanni," I tease, "share a juicy thigh with me, then I'll let you sample the pleasures of my figgy pudding." Giovanni easily relents at my irresistible offer. We devour the thigh. We relish the delights of my figgy pudding. We feel well satisfied.

Soon after, with great fanfare, Giovanni delivers the exquisitely roasted crane to Currado and his illustrious table of guests. I watch from behind a curtain. Currado brandishes the carving knife and begins to carve. Then he begins to frown,

"What the devil?" he exclaims, his frown deepening with rage, "Giovanni, you scoundrel, this bird is missing a leg." Though churning inside, Giovanni calmly replies, as I have carefully tutored him,

"But sire, a crane only has one leg."

Unwilling to engage in badinage with his cook in front of his sniggering guests, Currado curtly addresses Giovanni between clenched teeth,

"Early tomorrow morning, you and I shall go to the river, and there we shall see if the crane has one leg or two."

That night, Giovanni is aquiver with anxieties; what will his enraged master do to him when the truth is revealed in the morning?

"You worry too much," I laughingly chide him. Tenderly, I tell him exactly what he must say.

Early the next morning, they take mount and ride to the river, Currado on a fine stallion, Giovanni on an old nag. As they approach the river, they see a dozen cranes, standing in the water, all of them on one leg.

"There, you see, sire," mumbles Giovanni, with great trepidation, despite my tutoring, "all these cranes have only one leg."

Currado gives Giovanni an evil look, then turning to the cranes he calls out, "Boo!"

At once, all the cranes lower their other leg, take a few steps, and take off into the air.

"There, you see, you miserable wretch," Currado shouts, "that shows you, a crane has two legs."

"Yes indeed, sire." Giovanni humbly responds, then with rising assurance and glee,

"Yet, had you called out 'Boo!' at last night's crane, it would no doubt have lowered its other leg."

Currado, both apoplectic with rage and helpless with laughter, finally splutters out,

"Giovanni, you are right, that is what I should have done, and now, what a fine tale I have to tell at the dining table whenever we feast on crane."

So it was, for ever after, thanks to my quick wits, Giovanni could enjoy with me an abundance of crane's leg and copious figgy pudding, so soft and moist and sweet.

Source

This story is loosely based on the story *The Crane's Leg* from Giovanni Boccaccio's *The Decameron* (ca. 1353).

Reflections

Egalitarian Reflection

There is still a prevailing view that it's the man who initiates a relationship with a woman—the image of him on bended knee with flowers and a ring. To my mind it's tosh. It is by subtle hints, a trivial touch, and a casual compliment, with which a woman can quietly enchant a chosen man into thinking it's his idea. Anything other risks being oppressive, even abusive.

Your Psychological Reflection

Put yourself in the mind of a distinguished professional, assiduously and proficiently absorbed in his task. How aware might he be of a mere pastry cook? What might be his inner response when approached by a pastry cook? An affront to his dignity? Irritated by the distraction? A little unnerved? And, when this pastry cook has the audacity to flirt with him, "Let's share a thigh together"? Well, of course, the distinguished professional is scandalised at the very idea, yet I wonder what else might stir in his psyche, what do you imagine? Where is Giovanni in his psychospiritual development?

Turn your reflective imagination onto the mere pastry cook. How does she see herself? Rate herself? What fantasies does she have about the distinguished professional dominating the kitchen? How does she see herself in relation to this distinguished professional? How might it be for her were he to rebuff her? Where is Brunette in her psychospiritual development?

A distinguished professional and a mere pastry cook, where does the power lie? And why?

My Psychological Reflection

At the turning of the Wheel, a woman in a kitchen offers figgy pudding to a man. This is a woman infused with sexual potency, her feelings freely flowing, her body beautifully contained, a clear mind with an incisive wit, her vital spirit imbued with acute inner wisdom and intent, a woman who knows how to work her will. It was right to set the story in the first person; this is her magnificent story.

I sometimes find with couples that understanding, insight, and wisdom sit more comfortably on the shoulders of the woman than the man. I surmise that the woman is further along in her psychospiritual journey than he is, and at the same time she can see his potential. In the story, Giovanni has enough insight to know that being willing to be guided by Brunette is to his best advantage, beyond the benefits of figgy pudding.

This is not always so. However gently the woman might seek to guide the man, he might react by accusing her of being controlling. Feeling controlled invokes pre-personal feelings of low self-esteem, causing him to react with truculence. The woman may be so sure in her personal self conviction of what's best for the man, that feeling thwarted by his obduracy she becomes annoyed with him. In the context of couple therapy this kind of impasse is difficult to work with. I have found that couple therapy benefits from a judicious mix of couple sessions for working on the relationship and individual sessions to address phase-related issues.

What about Giovanni? A man who has perfected his trade and worked hard to win success and reputation, what more has life to offer? As Matthew Arnold (Dover Beach and Other Poems) wrote,

> For most men in a brazen prison live,
> Where, in the sun's hot eye,
> With heads bent o'er their toil, they languidly
> Their lives to some unmeaning taskwork give,
> Dreaming of naught beyond their prison wall.
> And as, year after year,
> Fresh products of their barren labour fall
> From their tired hands, and rest
> Never yet comes more near,
> Gloom settles slowly down over their breast.
> And while they try to stem
> The waves of mournful thought by which they are prest,
> Death in their prison reaches them,
> Unfreed, having seen nothing, still unblest.

Is this Giovanni? A dispirited conformist, obeying the rules, just a servant despite his reputation, dreaming of naught? What did you imagine might stir in his psyche? When a spirited, passionate pastry cook in a kitchen offers figgy pudding to him? It seems, serendipity arises, he comes to feel well satisfied, and not just by figgy pudding.

The Laydys of the Towne

> *'The Laydys of the Towne' is such a tasty tale. Moreover, much of what I shall quote, as the tale unfolds, comes from a contemporary journal written by Peter Clarke, clerk to Mr Craikenthorp, attorney at law in Penrith. This is folk history. Being a Lancashire lad from Preston, I am not unfamiliar with its Very Beautyfull Laydys, or perhaps I should say, I am familiar.*

As everything begins in the imagination,
healing begins in the imagination.

Synopsis

The Laydys of the Towne is a contemporary account of how the laydys found an imaginative way of bringing the Jacobite rebellion of 1715 to an end and thereby preventing widespread slaughter.

In the words of the Duke of Marlborough, of Blenheim fame, in overall command of Government forces, "the very beautyfull laydys of Preston and their courting and ffeasting" were the undoing of the Jacobites—not overlooking their cousins, the very beautyfull laydys of Lancaster.

The Story

Lancaster Laydys of the Towne

Men are prey to such delusions. Our great Parliamentarians thought the best way to choose a new Head of State was to scour the bloodlines of minor European royalty to find someone who professed the Protestant faith. Jacobites, on the other hand, embraced 'Mister Melancholy', 'King Over the Water' James Francis Stuart, who according to a disillusioned supporter, Viscount Bolingbroke, "dwelt in a maze of unrealities."

When Queen Anne died and non-English-speaking Georgie the Wurst was crowned King, the perspicacious populace exercised their sole form of political expression by pouring onto the streets in protest. The deluded Jacobites thought this meant the people supported James Stuart. On the strength of this they staged a rebellion.

The Earl of Mar raised the Stuart standard in Scotland. In Northumberland, the rising was led by the Earl of Derwentwater, Lord Widdrington, and Mr Thomas Foster, MP for the county. Derwentwater and Widdrington being Roman Catholics, they feared if either were chosen to lead the Jacobite forces, Protestant susceptibilities might be hurt. On this implausible basis, Protestant Thomas Foster was made General, despite his lack of military training or, as it turned out, acumen.

Widdrington had convinced Foster that, in Manchester, 20,000 impoverished younger sons of dispossessed Civil War Royalists had been forced to seek a livelihood in commerce and were ready to take up arms in the Jacobite cause. This conviction became the guiding illusion of Foster's campaign. Making its way south after assembling in Kelso, the small rebel army proclaimed James III as King of England at Penrith, Appleby, Kendal and Kirby Lonsdale, and in each town they collected excise duties due to the Crown and confiscated any arms and gunpowder they discovered. At Kendal, General Foster visited his godmother, Madame Belingham, who promptly boxed his ears and called him a rebel and popish tool.

The rebel army entered Lancaster in their ranks, with swords drawn, colours flying, drums beating and bagpipes playing. James III was proclaimed King. A search was made for arms, during which shopkeeper Samuel Satherwaite bestowed the only barrel of gunpowder to the town's well rather than sell it to the insurgents. A rebel Church of England minister, Mr William Paul, read Matins in the church, substituting 'King James' for 'King George' in the Book of Common Prayer.

Meanwhile, the 'laydys of the towne' prepared to entertain their guests. Stripping off their day clothes, they laced on tall-waisted stays, wide-fronted and narrow-backed, a loose gown of soft material with a skirt belling out over the hips, an open-fronted bodice with a richly decorated stomacher and a coordinating petticoat. The overall effect was of broad hips, narrow waist, erect posture, and high, full, firm breasts, très décolleté as Lancashire women say, the zenith of allure.

The women garnished their board as handsomely as their resplendent figures, as they laid out the fruits of Morecambe Bay, baked fluke, heaps of cockles and mussels, great tubs of shrimps oozing with warm butter, as well as whole baked salmon, pork chops, pheasant breasts, venison steaks, dishes of quaking pudding, shivering trifle, baked apples, fresh cream—and gigantic pots of Yorkshire tea.

Now the women were ready. In the afternoon, the 'laydys of the towne' invited the gentlemen soldiers to drink a dish of tea with them. The invitation was warmly received, and 'the gentlemen soldiers dressed and trimmed themselves up in their best cloathes for to drink a dish of tea with the laydys of this towne'. The women 'apeared in their best riging, and had their tea tables richly furnished for to entertain their new suitors'—and also to divert them.

The tea party was a singular, scintillating triumph. The gentlemen soldiers were utterly captivated by the flattering words and soft caresses of the 'very beautyfull laydys', enticing them away from all thought of conflict, but with glad hearts and full bellies they lost all appetite for affray, save for the swordplay of romance.

Until, at that climactic moment, Rev William Paul and General Foster strode in on heavy boots to declare a discourse about religion between William Paul and two papist priests to take place forthwith. Early the next morning, secure in Widdrington's promise of a Mancunian Jacobite host, General Foster led his army out of Lancaster—a town easy of defence with ready access by sea to sympathisers in France and Ireland—and on the road to poorly defensible Preston.

The Lancaster women were disappointed but not disheartened by the abrupt withdrawal of their suitors. They relayed an urgent message, faster than any army could travel, via Scotforth, Ellel, Scorton, Garstang, Barton, and Broughton to the women of Preston, warning them of the approach of the Jacobite army and urging them to be ready.

The Very Beautyfull Laydys of Preston

Preston was the metropolis of the County Palatine of Lancaster. Many county families kept a fine house in the town, which boasted a mild climate, a picturesque location on cliffs above the River Ribble, and ease of access from the whole of Lancashire. The leading gentry of the county flocked to Preston for the 'Winter Season', which was one long round of merriment, with costume balls, charades, rowdy routs, concerts, masques, and plays.

On a Wednesday evening in November, the Jacobite army arrived at Preston. The women of the town were ready. They greeted the gentlemen soldiers with open arms, even General Foster, whisking them away into a frenzied whirligig of entertainment, delight, and diversion. 'The very beautyfull laydys of Preston' were even more alluring than their Lancastrian cousins, their hips broader, their waists narrower, their posture more erect and tall, their breasts higher, more full, more firm, décolleté très généreux et plongeant as Preston women say, the peak of feminine perfection.

'The very beautyfull laydys' ply their suitors with fine wines, sweetmeats, tasty treats, and amorous morsels. They organise masked balls where they can take their swains gently by the hand and lead them to quiet arbours to reveal their secret pleasures.

The weariness of the gentlemen soldiers' long march from Scotland falls away, as they gleefully give themselves to this glittering life of dancing and laughter, of feasting and carousing, of amusement and amours. The urgency of the Jacobite cause gives way: lethargy and lassitude hold sway. As was remarked at the time, "The laydys in this toune are so very beautyfull and so richly atired, that the gentlemen soldiers from Wednesday to Saturday minded nothing but courting and ffeasting."

On Friday night Lord Derwentwater received a military despatch that a Government force of several thousand men under General Wills, only 12 miles away at Wigan, was about to march on Preston.

Derwentwater found General Foster upon his couch enjoying convivial entertainment. As Foster struggled to take in Derwentwater's news, his befuddled mind could grasp nothing to dislodge his belief in an illusory Mancunian mob. He waved aside the despatch and returned to his cordial couch.

Come Saturday morning, General Wills and his men were seen near Walton le Dale, close to the Ribble bridge. Barricades were belatedly and hastily erected. As General Wills' men approached the town, Highlanders at the barricade by the church on Churchgate offered a spirited defence, which held off the Government forces overnight, to the short-lived rejoicing of the defenders.

There was further skirmishing the following day, with, in all, about three hundred casualties, mostly Government soldiers, but by Monday morning General Wills' forces had encircled the town and held it in a vice. To the chagrin of the brave Highlanders, who wanted to fight their way out, the Earl of Derwentwater surrendered, and Jacobite hopes lay in the dust.

"The very beautyfull laydys of Preston and their courting and ffeasting" had proved to be the undoing of the Jacobite rebellion.

Sources

Berry, A. J. (1912); Clarke, Peter (Written 1715) and Paton, Henry M. A. (Ed., 1893); Fishwick, Henry (1894); Hird, Frank (1912), Volume I.

Reflections

Psychological Reflection, Egalitarian as well

This deceptively simple story draws a sharp distinction between 'men', intent on marching, plundering, grandiose discourses, proud proclamations, and aggression, on the basis of a flawed analysis of the public mood, and 'women', with clear intent on putting an end to conflict by luring 'men' to enjoy simple humane pleasures, feasting, fellowship, supping tea, partying, and amours.

And this was 300 years before neuroscience research (Iain McGilchrist *The Master and His Emissary*, 2009) revealed the differing functions of left and right hemispheres, or in the terms of the story 'men' and 'women'.

The right and left brains have distinctly differing modes of thought. The functions of the right brain include the human qualities of insight, intuition, and creativity; feelings and passions; sense of self; relationships; empathy; compassion; and not least humour. The functions of the left brain include the use of language in order to articulate: understanding of the construction of known objects; analysis of things into their component parts; conclusions from analysing real-life situations; as well as anger, aggression, and disgust.

As we know, beneath the simple story there often lies a deeper, complex story, a psychological story.

Assertive of their personal conviction that James Stuart is the rightful king, the leaders of the rebellion arrive at their flawed analysis of the public mood. Unencumbered by such conviction, the laydys of Lancaster's analysis is that the rebellion will lead to catastrophe and widespread slaughter of innocent folk. Their intuitive response is to create a plan to subvert the rebellion and thereby prevent loss of life. The laydys first use their left brain mode of thought to analyse the situation, then they use their right brain mode of thought to create a response that expresses qualities of relationship and compassion. They create a synthesis of the differing modes of thought.

If only we human beings could learn to synthesise left- and right-brain modes of thought, our species, and many other species, would be safer and more secure.

From the perspective of psychospiritual development, the rebellion leaders, with their fixed conviction, display the second phase, personal, whilst the laydys display the third phase, transpersonal.

From the perspective of the dynamic portrayal of soul—all energy being sexual energy—the rebellion leaders are portrayed as deploying their energy in grandiosity and aggression, whilst the laydys are portrayed as deploying their energy with humour, verve, and spirit in their unconcealed sexuality.

Demeter and Persephone

The irruption of Baubo, Goddess of Rude Jokes, into the classical myth of 'Demeter and Persephone' is divertingly transformative; ribaldry is an epiphany for Demeter, undoing her dark mood, affording courage and cunning to trounce her arrogant, errant spouse. When goddesses get together, drollery resounds.

If you know any of Baubo's rude jokes, please share them with me.
The story is the healer; the story touches the Soul.

Synopsis

Hades abducts Demeter's daughter Persephone with the connivance of Zeus. Hades carries off Persephone to be Queen of the Underworld. After learning what had happened to her daughter, Demeter is consumed by anger and grief. In her anger, she brings famine. In deep grief, she wanders from place to place in the guise of an old woman until she meets Baubo, whose bawdy jokes touch her Soul and restore her Spirit. She confronts Zeus and threatens him with perpetual austerity unless he has Persephone restored to her, which incidentally creates Spring.

The Story

The immortal gods lived upon Mount Olympus. Lacking any other occupation, they spent their time making trouble and playing nasty tricks on one another. And, of course, drinking nectar and eating ambrosia—a kind of rice pudding—which they liked so much they couldn't do without it.

Demeter was an exceptional exception. She was the Goddess of Harvest and Fertility, devoting her life to the nurture of humankind by ensuring that the land was fertile, the crops were abundant, the fruit was plentiful, and the people were content.

Persephone was the daughter of Demeter and the great Zeus, God of Sky. Were you to meet Persephone, youthful, breathtakingly statuesque, graceful, fair of face, and tall of stature, with her legs long and shapely, you would think her a goddess—which indeed she was, the Goddess of Grain. Persephone spent her days assisting her mother in her work, ensuring that the crops grew tall, bent over with copious grain. Demeter loved her daughter to distraction.

Hades was the God of the Underworld. There was little to light the darkness of Hades' world, yet he had taken a shine to Persephone, lusting after her with an obsessive urgency that caught the warped attention of Zeus. A plot was hatched. One day, while Persephone was picking pansies and lilies in a glade, Hades abducted her, with the connivance of Zeus, and bore her off to be Queen of the Underworld.

Demeter was filled with grief, anger, and dread and, unaware of his complicity, appealed to Zeus for help to return Persephone to her. Zeus simply returned a sneering grin, a sure sign of his collusion in the plot. Demeter was beside herself with rage. In her rage, she stopped the crops from growing, and there was famine throughout the land. But on Mount Olympus the gods toasted Zeus' prank with gallons of nectar and copious bowls of ambrosia.

Demeter was heartbroken. She took the gown and guise of an old woman, and in deep grief she wandered from town to town until she reached Eleusis. There she met Baubo, Goddess of Rude Jokes, in the palace of the king.

Baubo's face was upon her belly. Her breasts were bulging eyes. She had a protruding belly-button nose. Laughter lines spread out from her wide, smiling slit of a mouth, with its full lips. She had a ginger beard. Staring at Baubo's startling looks, Demeter almost smiled.

Baubo told bawdy jokes. Jokes I wouldn't tell my grandmother.

{Alas, I could find no record of these jokes. I scoured the libraries of the world—British Library, Library of Congress, Royal Library of Antioch, Imperial Library of Constantinople, Library of Pergamum—nothing! Until finally I unearthed this one in the Great Library of Alexandria:}

> **A Special Gift**. For decades, statues of a male and a female god face each other in a city park, looking longingly into one another's eyes, well, more of a stony stare, for year after year.
>
> One day, Hermes flies in from Olympus.
>
> "You've been such fine exemplars of the gods," Hermes said, "that I've come to give you a special gift. I'm going to bring you back to life for thirty minutes so you can do anything you desire." And with a clap of hands Hermes brings the statues to life. The two approach each other, shyly at first, then dash for the bushes. There come sounds of merriment, giggling, laughter, and the shaking of bushes. Fifteen minutes later the statues emerge from the bushes, cracking up these statues are, laughing their heads off, with wide smiles of delight on their faces.
>
> "You still have fifteen minutes," says Hermes, with a wink. Smiling even more broadly the female statue turns to the male statue and says,
>
> "Great, only this time you hold the pigeon down and I'll shit on it's head."

Listening to Baubo's bawdy jokes, Demeter began to smile, then grin, titter, giggle, chuckle, snigger, laugh, chortle, hoot, snort, guffaw, fall about. Then, she rose up with lifted spirits and new heart. She went straight to Olympus and faced up to Zeus,

"Look here Zeus, this is how it is, you're going to help me restore Persephone. Otherwise, as I'm the Goddess of Harvest and Fertility, the land will stay barren. There'll be no flowers, so no nectar. There'll be no rice, so no ambrosia. You'll suffer terrible withdrawal symptoms. And, as you're immortal, you'll suffer terrible withdrawal symptoms for the whole of eternity. Ha! So, what are going to do about it?"

Zeus saw he had no choice but to send Hermes, messenger of the gods, to tell Hades to release Persephone. Hermes asked Persephone what she had eaten in the Underworld.

"Not a thing," she replied, "except, six pomegranate seeds." Hermes rolled his eyes and told Persephone,

"For each pomegranate seed, you must spend a month every year underground. You'll prepare the ground for this new-fangled 'season' called 'Spring'."

So it was that Persephone remained Queen of the Underworld as well as Goddess of Grain and Spring.

Source

Demeter and Persephone is a Greek myth, part of the Eleusinian Mysteries. Wikipedia tells us: At a certain spot along the processional route to Eleusis, the people shouted obscenities in commemoration of Baubo, an old woman who, by cracking dirty jokes, had made Demeter smile as she mourned the loss of her daughter.

Reflections

Egalitarian Reflection

Though the myth of *Demeter and Persephone* is told with a light touch to entertain a public audience, the story's subject is abhorrent. It's a horror story. Zeus rapes his sister Demeter, thereby begetting his daughter Persephone. Subsequently, he conspires in the abduction and rape of his daughter Persephone by his brother Hades. So it's not only rape, it's incestuous rape, a yet further life-distorting injury.

Demeter and Persephone being set in a rape culture, the tale is acutely relevant to our contemporary culture; the Rape Crisis website reports that one in four adult women, totalling 6.54 million women, have been raped or sexually assaulted. And that's just England and Wales; it's a worldwide scourge. The Rape Crisis website, as well as providing much pertinent information, describes common myths about rape, sexual assault, sexual abuse, and other types of sexual violence causing serious harm, together with the true facts in each case.

Your Psychological Reflection

What feelings arose for you on first reading the above myth? What do you feel now, after reading the Egalitarian Reflection? I invite you to enjoy reading the myth again, with its light touch, while keeping firmly in mind the Hadean dark beneath and suffering the tension between the two.

My Psychological Reflection

After Persephone's abduction and rape, Demeter is overwhelmed by grief. Not knowing where to turn, she wanders aimlessly from town to town in the garb of an old woman, emotionally as barren as her land, barren even of happy memories of her daughter, consumed as she is by grief.

It takes Baubo's ribald humour for Demeter to make a psychological shift, enabling her to differentiate from her feelings of grief and to restore the integration of her whole being—feelings, body, mind, and spirit—liberating her anger and mustering the energy and moral strength she needs to contend with conniving Zeus.

Differentiation and integration describe the process of grieving: differentiation from fusion with bitter memories of death and loss and integration with warm and tender memories of one who has passed. Differentiation and integration also describe, for a therapist, a guide for psychotherapeutic work with a grieving client.

There are moments with a distressed client when, quite naturally, their tearful face will light up and they will utter a titter, easing the ache and lifting the spirit. Humour, a humane quality of the right brain (McGilchrist, 2009).

From her bright, gratifying life tending the crops, Persephone is borne off and sexually abused, finding herself in darkness. Her life will never be the same. Although she gains freedom from the dark, the desiccated seeds of darkness always lure her back.

For any abused woman or child, life will never be the same. When someone is sexually abused, something lovely and precious, such as innocence, is taken away, and something bleak and weakening, commonly shame, is put in its place. The sexually abused woman in the therapy room needs us, in our role as therapist, to hold the woman's innocence in imagination for her until she can take it back.

Defiant Saxon Queens

The next two stories are about historical characters, Cynethryth Queen of the Mercians and Queen Emma of Normandy. I know, I know, Emma of Normandy wasn't a Saxon queen, but why ruin a good title over a detail. Anyway, she did marry the Saxon King Æthelred, and she was defiant.

Both Cynethryth and Emma employ their sexual wiles, though to differing ends. There is such a sharp contrast between Queen Emma, calmly exercising her will, and Cynethryth, driven by her history.

According to German philosopher Walter Benjamin, "History is written by the victors." So, history has an illusive quality. All the same, on my word of honour as a storyteller, the next two stories are unvarnished truth—though not without a certain interpretational flourish—and my fingers are uncrossed to prove it. Well, they are now.

Cynethryth Queen of the Mercians

Floating in from a murky past, a Frankish girl used her sexual wiles to become one of the most prominent women of the Saxon period. And one of the most ruthless.

The rise of Queen Cynethryth must be one of the singularly strangest tales in the history of monarchy. To mark her singularity, Cynethryth is the only Anglo-Saxon queen to have had coins issued in her name, and when Charlemagne wrote to his English counterparts, he wrote jointly to King Offa and Queen Cynethryth, affording them equal status.

After the death of her husband, Cynethryth became Abbess of a monastery at Cookham in Berkshire. The site of the monastery was only discovered and excavated in 2021.

The story is the healer.

Synopsis

For her ‘crimes’, a Frankish girl is set adrift in an open boat. She is washed up on the Welsh coast, where she is brought before King Offa of Mercia. She skilfully wields her wiles upon King Offa to become Queen of Mercia. With her sharp wits and wicked nature, she single-handedly adds the Kingdom of East Anglia to their domains.

The Story

A Frankish girl was set adrift in an open boat, as punishment for her crimes, at the mercy of winds and tides. The winds and tides were merciful, for they washed her up on the Welsh coast. The boat may have been caught by the Severn bore, carrying her upriver and fetching her up on a Welsh shore close to the Kingdom of Mercia. She was rescued by the King of Mercia’s steward and brought before Offa, King of Mercia.

Offa was moved by her beauty and her plaintive tale: her Frankish nobleman father had desired to wed her and had even appealed for permission from the Pope, but she had refused him. As an innocent girl, whose only crime was to protect her virtue, he had her cast adrift, weeping and forlorn, in an open boat.

When King Offa married her, she took the name Cynethryth, styling herself after the daughters of a previous King of Mercia, King Penda. She was now Queen of the Mercians.

When King Offa was to be visited by King Ethelbert of East Anglia, with an eye to marry one of Offa's daughters, Cynethryth saw her chance for further mischief,

"Offa, my lord and my love, here's your God-given good fortune to seize the Kingdom of East Anglia. You know, you've always wanted to." Offa responded,

"What wickedness are you thrusting into my head? Perish the thought," with a wicked smirk on his lips and his tongue thrust into his cheek.

Cynethryth made arrangements for their guest, a quiet chamber, with rich hangings, a king-sized bed, and an irresistibly comfortable, sumptuously curtained easy chair, knowing that Ethelbert would cast himself into the chair before entering his rest. His eternal rest as it happens. Cynethryth had had her servants dig a deep pit with the chair atop. Later, with a sigh of pleasure, Ethelbert fell into the chair and—Surprise! Surprise!—fell into the pit, where the servants smothered the King with the finest goose-feather pillows, eiderdowns, and shovels of earth.

Shortly after, King Offa annexed the Kingdom of East Anglia, thanks to the inventive villainy of his beloved queen, Queen Cynethryth of Mercia and East Anglia. After King Offa died, Queen Cynethryth spent her closing years in a monastery as its Abbess.

Reflections

Your Psychological Reflection

Be you a man or a woman, what would it be like for you to have a highly sexed predatory woman like Cynethryth in your therapy room, or a highly sexed predatory man come to that? How willing might you be to work with them? How would you work with them? What might you discern about their character and their psychological development?

How do you fit Cynethryth on the Medicine Wheel? What are her Feelings? How are these expressed in her Body? What impressions does her Mind receive from her Feelings, her Body, and her surroundings? How would you describe her Spirit, how she presents herself to the world? What might be the Soul experience of herself?

My Psychological Reflection

Whilst a person has the Will to survive in the world, the ego still runs on rails, restricted to the tracks laid down in their assimilated 'way of being', with its system of values, beliefs, attitudes, aspirations, and their false beliefs about themselves: I'm not good enough; I'm unloveable; I don't need anybody…

According to the UK Office for National Statistics, a disproportionate number of 23- to 24-year-olds who have received custodial or non-custodial convictions had been classed as vulnerable during childhood, giving some indication of the 'way of being' they assimilated in a child-unfriendly family environment.

There can be no assumption that a mature ego, a survival self, is emotionally frail or benign. One successful business leader's mindset, assimilated from a fiercely ambitious father and honed over a lifetime of merciless dealings, was severe and simple: it's a jungle out there, rules are made to be broken, winning is everything.

Cynethryth is neither emotionally frail nor benign. Psychologically fused with her untold cruel history, she has no choice but to act out of that history. Though she has gained a measure of mature ego, a survival self, she has done so at a cost. She is selfish, seductive, ruthless, and wily, driven to use her sexuality as a way to survive, perpetually seeking to advance and enhance her power and prestige, without—I surmise—ever feeling safe.

Queen Emma's Ordeal By Fire

Defeated in battle, a woman gathers her sexual allure, her skilful will, and her moral strength to overcome her adversary. Later, falsely accused of sexual infidelity and facing an ordeal by fire, she further demonstrates her courage and spiritual power.

The story is the healer
and serves as a container for each listener's Soul energy.

Synopsis

To maintain her power and fortune, after King Cnut had successfully invaded her land, Queen Emma adroitly seduced Cnut into making her his queen. Later, after a period of uncertainty, her son Edward becomes king, but with relations strained with her son, who had come under the influence of Robert Abbot of Jumièges and had made him Archbishop of Canterbury, Emma's life is in danger. Robert is an ambitious, jealous, and unscrupulous prelate, and for him it is intolerable that Emma should have any influence with her son. He accuses her of having had sex with Ælfwine, Bishop of Winchester, and contrives to have her face an ordeal by fire. She is to prove her own innocence and that of the now dead Bishop, by stepping over nine red-hot ploughshares unscathed.

The Story

Cnut, son of Sweyn Forkbeard, once King of Denmark, Norway and England, invaded the land. King Æthelred and Queen Emma held out in London against Cnut's offensive. Within the year, however, Æthelred was dead, and Emma was holding out alone against the forces of Cnut.

Power, politics, passion and piety characterised this turbulent life of Emma of Normandy, twice Queen Consort and mother of two kings of England.

Queen Emma was the second wife of King Æthelred. Though she had been made to use the name of King Æthelred's first wife, Ælfgifu, on formal occasions, in the bargain she struck with Æthelred this humiliation was weightily counterbalanced by receiving extensive lands which had belonged to King Æthelred's mother, Queen Ælfthryth. Queen Emma continued Queen Ælfthryth's pious practice of largesse towards the clergy and religious houses.

When Cnut went to parley with Emma for a kingdom, expecting her to plead for life and liberty for herself and her sons, he came away with more than he had bargained for. He gained not only the Kingdom of England but also a passionate wife and powerful political ally.

When Emma went to parley with Cnut, she had in mind an inventive twist to her fortunes: to swap the cockpit of conflict for the marriage bed. She employed all her passionate allure and political guile to seduce her adversary, thereby retaining her political power, securing the safety of her sons, and acquiring a worthy lover to share her bed. The love match between Cnut the Great and Queen Emma lasted nearly 20 years until Cnut's death, and they had one son, Cnut's heir Harthacnut.

When Cnut the Great died, Harold Harefoot, Cnut's illegitimate son by his former 'handfast' wife, seized the kingdom while Harthacnut was busy fighting in Scandinavia. Emma's sons, Edward and Alfred, escaped to Normandy, and Emma took refuge in Bruges with the Count of Flanders, where she commissioned a treatise, *In Praise of Queen Emma*.

Back at the English court, Harold Harefoot had died, and though Harthacnut had been declared king and Edward had been sworn in as his heir, Harthacnut's grip on power remained fragile. By circulating *In Praise of Queen Emma*, Emma sought to garner political support for her sons and herself, successfully as it turned out, by shamelessly and cleverly presenting history in a way which placed Cnut, herself, and her sons in the best possible light.

A surprising woman, when Harthacnut died she supported Magnus, King of Norway and Denmark, as King of England rather than her son Edward. We can only speculate why she favoured, over her own blood, a 16-year-old lad with light blond hair, regular features and a light complexion, who was quick-witted, generous, and a brave warrior. For once her machinations failed, and Edward, later Edward the Confessor, became king.

Whatever Emma's reason for favouring Magnus, it strained her relationship with her son and left her in disgrace in the eyes of his court. With restored perspicacity, she chose to make her home at her manor in the Berkshire village of Wargrave. This avoided embarrassment to her son by creating some distance from his court. At the same time, it allowed her reasonable access to him in London or Winchester via the old London-Silchester-Winchester road. Despite his ambivalence towards her as his mother, she knew the king still valued her political insights. She also knew he was malleable, and in this way she could retain her political influence.

This is the quality of the woman, determined, inventive, surprising, and with a passionate nature, who was to face an ordeal by fire at the behest of Robert, Archbishop of Canterbury.

Robert was a Norman. He had been Abbot of Jumièges and had met and befriended Edward in his long exile in Normandy during Cnut's reign. He had accompanied Edward on his return to England to become king on Harthacnut's death and was one of Edward's closest advisers. Robert was ruthlessly ambitious, his crowning achievement to date being to have Edward appoint him as Archbishop of Canterbury despite the cathedral chapter's election of a different candidate. Robert bitterly resented any other influence on the king but his own and had driven Lord Godwin, another close adviser, into exile by accusing him of plotting to kill the king.

For Robert, therefore, the influence of King Edward's mother, Queen Emma, could not be tolerated. Moreover, this fastidious, celibate monk felt a profound distaste for women in general, and for this woman in particular, for her worldliness and flamboyant allure.

She had to go. But how was he to persuade the king to get rid of his own mother? Her support for Magnus was not sufficient to indict her, for she had otherwise been fully supportive of her son throughout his life, but it gave him a clue to her downfall: her passionate nature would destroy her.

Robert advised the king,

"I deeply regret to tell thee, sire, Ælfwine, Bishop of Winchester until his death three years ago, was overly intimate with thy mother, Queen Emma. As Archbishop of Canterbury it is my holy duty to ask thee to have Queen Emma prove her innocence, and also, as Ælfwine is no longer here to prove himself, she must prove his innocence at the same time. I am deeply saddened, sire, to have to bring these tidings." Thus did Robert seek to persuade the king to subject his mother to an ordeal by fire.

The king ordered Emma's lands and property to be confiscated, and she was sent to a nunnery, Wherwell Abbey. Reflecting on this sudden reversal of her fortunes, Emma realised how, by isolating her malleable son, Robert was a threat not only to herself but also to the king and his kingdom. In her response to this threat, Emma's political acumen, passion, piety, and capacity to surprise were to attain a new level.

Emma appealed for support to bishops whom she trusted. When the bishops rallied to Emma's support, this pushed Robert into risking stronger language in the presence of the king,

"She is a wild thing, not a woman. She called her slimy lover Christ the Lord," and worse words he uttered against her until the king consented to the ordeal by fire.

Though his face remained impassive, Robert was satisfied and even felt a little pleasure in his shrivelled heart at having trounced his rival, Queen Emma, so easily.

For the ordeal by fire, Queen Emma was to walk over nine ploughshares heated in the fire until they were red hot and placed on the pavement of Winchester Cathedral. As Robert dictated, four ploughshares were to prove her innocence and five to prove the innocence of Bishop Ælfwine, a double purgation. If Queen Emma were to walk over all nine red-hot ploughshares unscathed, then her innocence and that of Ælfwine would be proved, but if her feet were burned, then she would be proved guilty and condemned to death.

Queen Emma spent the night before her ordeal in prayer to St Swithun, who had been Bishop of Winchester in the time of King Ælfred the Great and was renowned for having overseen the rebuilding of Winchester's East Gate Bridge over the River Itchen. When visiting the bridge to review the work, St Swithun had met a poor woman in great distress, having dropped and broken her basket of eggs. He lightly plucked the basket from the ground and handed it back to her with his blessing, then carried on with his work. When she looked in the basket, to her joy the eggs had all been made whole.

As Queen Emma prayed, she brought this prosaic miracle to mind and held St Swithun in her heart with such pious fervour that the saint came to her, saying,

"I am Swithun whom thou hast invoked. Fear not, the fire shall do thee no hurt."

Early the next morning, a fire was lit in the nave of Winchester's Cathedral Church of St Swithun, and the nine ploughshares were placed in the fire until they were red hot and ready to be placed on the pavement when King Edward the Confessor and his whole court were assembled with the cathedral clergy and Archbishop Robert.

Queen Emma enters the cathedral blindfolded, led by the Bishop of Winchester. With the reassuring words of the cathedral's patron saint in her heart, she utters an invocation,

"Oh God, who didst save Susannah from the malice of the wicked elders, save me, I humbly entreat thee."

Led by the bishop, she trips lightly across the pavement of the nave, so lightly she feels that were she walking upon eggs, they would not break beneath her feet. Turning to the bishop, she asks,

"When shall we come to the ploughshares?"

"Why, ma'am," he replies in humble amazement, falling upon his knees before her, "By St Swithun, thou hast stepped upon them already and thou art unharmed. This miracle proves thine innocence and that of the blessed Ælfwine."

King Edward the Confessor is mortified at having subjected his mother to such a cruel and humiliating torment, and in that moment, contemplating her demeanour throughout this ordeal, he feels he sees and appreciates her qualities for the very first time. He casts himself at her feet in repentance and pleads for her forgiveness. He throws off his robes, tears off his shirt, exposing his back to the lash, and submits to atoning stripes from Queen Emma and the Bishop of Winchester. Emma's lands and property are restored.

In gratitude to St Swithun for her deliverance, Queen Emma gave nine of her manors, one for each ploughshare, to the See of Winchester. One of these was her manor of Wargrave.

Robert had overreached himself. By her self-control and calm demeanour throughout her ordeal, Emma had exposed Robert's overweening and ruthless ambition. He was deposed from his archbishopric at a royal council, stripped of all his personal property, declared an outlaw, and banished to Normandy, where he died soon afterwards, a broken man.

Note

According to Berkshire folklore, Queen Emma lived for part of her life in Wargrave, survived an ordeal by fire at Winchester after having been accused by Archbishop Robert of infidelity with the deceased Bishop Ælfwine, and in gratitude to St Swithun gave her Wargrave manor, along with eight more, to the Bishop of Winchester.

Source

Gray, Rosemary (Ed.) (c1986) *The Book of Wargrave*, Wargrave Local History Society, p. 183.

First published in Berkshire Folk Tales (David England and Tina Bilbé, 2013).

Reflections

Your Psychological Reflection

Emma is a new client. She is in crisis, telling you she has lost everything: her husband, her home, her possessions, and her standing in the world. Even her life and liberty are threatened. What is your first reaction? Can she afford to pay me? What really is the issue bringing her into therapy? How would you begin to work with her? Where would your focus be? How would you assess her psychologically, at each stage: Pre-personal, Personal, Transpersonal? Where is her Centre of Gravity? What might you look for in her that could help her to help herself?

Turning to the tale, I invite you to reflect on the Dynamic Portrayal of Emma's Soul. Emma is passionate in her Feelings, yet despite dread fears over the threat to her life and liberty, her Body contains these fears, her Mind remains focused and creative, and she portrays considerable Spirit. Seducing Cnut the Great may be a tactic to get out of a hole or a strategy of partnership with a worthy lover, a man she can admire, with whom she bears a king, and with whom she remains loyal for 20 years.

I invite you to wonder, how much is the relationship between Emma and Cnut a strategic alliance or a love match? Both? Reflect on Emma's Sexuality—in the comprehensive sense described in *A Portrait of Soul*—how much is her sexuality in full flow as the Wheel turns?

My Psychological Reflection

Not only has Queen Emma lost her king, her kingdom, and her power, but also her life and liberty are threatened. Facing catastrophe, this woman reveals her evolved psychology in her moral strength, personal power, and skilful will. Queen Emma has already shown herself not to be one to act impulsively or for short-term survival gain. Keeping a cool head, she reflects strategically on the options she has in the best interests of herself and her kingdom. She chooses to enchant Cnut and become his queen. Such a smart turnaround in her fortunes! She saves the kingdom for herself and her son and keeps her title as Queen Emma.

Later, when her reputation and life are threatened by the ruthlessly ambitious Archbishop, she remains courageous and resolute, willing to walk through fire to affirm and maintain her integrity, and again she wins the day.

The Abbess' Coif

Warning! *This tale should only be read after the nine o'clock watershed. It contains writing that may offend.*

For some men, in the past and even in the present, controlling or withholding the marriage of daughters is used as a form of oppression, as in this story.

I submitted this story for the Story Competition at Slough Writers Group, a fantastic, talented group that has met weekly for over 25 years. A panel of outside judges came to offer their feedback and give us the results. Their comments were considered and fair. When it came to my story, the chair of judges said, "This story has divided opinion." One of the men on the panel, it turned out, was a contributor to the Convent of the Sacred Heart of Mary.[1] *Oops! Well, at least the panel's opinion wasn't unanimous.*

The right story holds up a mirror to the listener's existential experience, and it is this which brings healing and transformation.

Synopsis

To avoid the cost of a marriage dowry, a nobleman consigns his daughter to a religious order of nuns. Far from submissively embracing her confinement, she embraces a young gallant and transforms the religious house into a house of some renown.

Egalitarian Reflection

The point of *The Abbess' Coif* story is that it takes moral strength, wit, wisdom, and courage embodied in her sexuality for a woman to survive and thrive in a sexually repressive environment. The judge in the above anecdote misses the point of the story, being caught up in outrage and moral judgement rather than in empathy and artistic appraisal.

Nicola Miller, one of the most experienced people working with former female school boarders, writes about young women in the 21st century who are boarding school survivors:

Girls are left with a deep distrust of their own womanhood. Not only do they feel unloved, rejected, but they also reject themselves. How can they hope to feel sexy, loveable, and whole as they struggle with such deep feelings of distrust and resentment of their mothers, whom they needed so badly to present a person with whom to identify.

Further information about Boarding School Survivors is available at www.boar dingschoolsurvivors.co.uk/

The Story

Long, long ago in Lombardy, the Abbey had an unenviable reputation for pure and holy living and the strictness and austerity of its rule. As well as for the quality of its inmates; marriage dowries being at a premium, it was cheaper for noblemen to endow their daughters as Brides of Christ. One such was Isabetta, a young woman of exquisite beauty of face and form.

One day, Isabetta was being visited by her brother and conversing with him through a grill. He was accompanied by a fine, young gallant. When this youth and Isabetta lighted upon each other, their eyes flashed with undisguised passion and desire.

The brother excused himself to attend the earth closet, giving the pair the opportunity to arrange an assignation. Isabetta disclosed to the gallant a secret way by which he might gain access to her cell, which he did that very night.

Isabetta cast off her coif and wimple, lifted her rude habit over her head, and let her simple white shift shimmy to the ground. She stood brazenly before the gallant clad in nought but her nun's black stockings and hobnailed boots. The gallant divested himself likewise.

Moving towards Isabetta, he ran his fingers through her soft curls. With his other hand he gently stroked her hair. Truth to tell, after an unconscionable time of disavowed celibacy, Isabetta was sadly unpractised in the art of love. But the gallant soon licked her into shape.

Thus, night after night the hours 'twixt compline and prime passed in passion and joy.

Alas, the gallant was observed in his secret entry to Isabetta's cell by scheming and jealous nuns. They plotted to expose Isabetta and bring her to shame and ignominy. One night, soon after the gallant had slipped into Isabetta's cell, these jealous nuns beat upon the Abbess' chamber door, calling out, "Up madam, up, Isabetta has a youth in her cell."

Now, as it happened, each night the Abbess had carried into her chamber a large chest believed to contain a holy relic, the very bones of St Bernard of Clairvaux, that she might spend the night upon her knees, bowing in reverence before the body of this heavenly man. Indeed, this was partly true, save that the heavenly body towards which she bowed was that of a young and eager priest.

In fact, at the very moment those jealous nuns were beating upon the Abbess' chamber door, the mortal remains of St Bernard of Clairvaux were being gnawed by the Abbey's shepherd bitch, later to be immortalised as St Lassie.

Disturbed in her oblations by the jealous nuns, the Abbess, scrabbling in the dark for her clothing, inadvertently put on her head the young priest's medieval Y-fronts.

{We need to introduce a fashion note here. The said Y-fronts had appealing side fringes reflecting the Y-motif. The whole ensemble was presented in scarlet and puce, these being ecclesiastical colours. Such attire was considered de rigueur for any ambitious priest eager to rise in the ecclesiastical hierarchy. Which the young priest achieved with the Abbess several times a night.}

The jealous nuns, consumed by lascivious thoughts and agog to witness Isabetta's antics with her lover, paid no heed to the Abbess' un-canonical headgear. Still attired in her nun's black stockings and hobnailed boots, Isabetta was dragged into the chapter house to stand before the Abbess and the whole lewdly gaping assembly to account for her flouting of the Abbey's strict rule.

The Abbess was much put out by so abrupt a coitus interruptus and took it out on the girl, berating her roundly for such disgraceful and abominable conduct, sullying the reputation of the Abbey for its pure and holy living and the strictness and austerity of its rule.

The young nun, likewise, was put out by so abrupt an interruptus. She felt more chagrin than shame, less guilt than exasperation, and was swollen with unsatisfied desire. Looking the Abbess in the face, she addressed her boldly,

"Madam, 'twere well thou should'st tie up thy coif afore upbraiding me further."

"What coif, thou lewd woman?" spluttered the Abbess, "Hast thou the effrontery to jest with me at such a time?"

"Prithee," quoth Isabetta, "tie up thy coif, then sayeth whatsoever thou pleaseth to me."

Hearing this exchange, the assembled nuns began to turn their lustful eyes away from Isabetta towards the Abbess. Gasps ran around the chapter house, rising to titters, chuckles, laughs, and belly laughs which rocked the chapter house—and the plumper nuns—to their very foundations. The Abbess' face turned as scarlet and puce as her elegant headgear. Afterwards, the Abbey's rule was much relaxed, and—though for Isabetta her dalliance with the young gallant thus lost much of its allure—the Abbey gained great renown amongst the noble young women in those parts.

Source

This story is loosely based on the story *The Abbess' Coif* from Giovanni Boccaccio's *The Decameron.*

Reflections

Your Psychological Reflection

"This story has divided opinion." So, ask yourself, what is my opinion? How do I experience it? What do I receive? What feelings? What thoughts? Reflections? Intuitions? Take your time. Where do my sympathies lie with the characters in the story? What are my attitudes to issues of sexuality? If the woman in my therapy room is Isabetta, existing in a sexually repressive situation, or raising a delicate sexual issue, how shall I work with her?

The main characters in the story are Isabetta and the Abbess—not forgetting St Lassie. Ask yourself, what can I learn about them in regard to their Portrayal of Soul: Feelings, Body, Mind, Spirit, and Sexuality, the expanding of Consciousness and Will?

My Psychological Reflection

"I've been torn from my home and family. I've been imprisoned with a bunch of women. I have to wear coarse clothes and scratchy nun's stockings. I should be wed, I'm old enough, my body aches. We sisters speak in whispers, such talk, such titters. I see a boy through the grille, my bowels turn over, such an urge, a surge. I didn't need to think about it. I didn't think about it. Now, here he is in my cell. I feel nervous, my first time. I get over it quick enough."

The Abbess' Coif paints a picture of repression, denial, and hypocrisy that has blighted women's expression of sexual feelings for millennia. Yet, locking Isabetta away, only allowing her to speak to men through a grill, doesn't prevent her from having sexual feelings or seizing an opportunity to satisfy them; for Isabetta, her undisguised passion and desire are far stronger than the strictness and austerity of any religious or moral rule.

This story has divided opinion about passion and desire in young women being far stronger than the strictness and austerity of any religious or moral rule or parental sanction. So, 'how to keep young women safe?' Isabetta is locked up in a nunnery. In some communities, observance of rules governing sexual conduct is strictly applied. A tactic last century was to weaponise fear and shame by treating 'fallen women' with brutality, denying them pain relief in childbirth, with cruelty and oppression reaching its apogee in the Magdalene Laundries, while letting 'fallen men' off scot-free. A Victorian approach was denial, only men have sexual feelings, or only men are entitled to them, so men are a danger, and women, who need to be chaperoned in their presence, lest a woman's reputation be sullied by association, an affront to men as well as women. A Victorian dame, counselling her daughter on the eve of marriage, "Yes, I know it's awful, my dear, but do as I did, just shut your eyes and think of England." How do you react to this anecdote?

All of these approaches to 'keeping young women safe' continue to be employed, even in the Western world with its fairly liberal sexual culture. I suggest 'keeping young women safe' is a wrong premise. On the contrary, we need to encourage young people to take responsibility for themselves and to give them the support and information they need to take their own life decisions.

As therapists, helping clients to take their own life decisions is what we do. In our role as therapists, we remain conscious that our role is neither to offer solutions from our own history nor from our own analysis, much less to take a moral stance, but to engage with our client in soulmaking, a mutual imaginative dialogue that is supporting him or her to find moral strength and courage in the expanding of Spirit and deepening of Soul. Early in my counselling work, I took a sexually abused woman client to supervision. My supervisor said, unless you deepen the work with this client, she'll leave. Soon after, she left. What effective therapy means for me now is that both I and my client experience in the work the expanding of Spirit and deepening of Soul.

Sir Gawain and the Green Knight

Though called 'Sir Gawain and the Green Knight', the tale is really about courtly love and the pursuit of courtly love by the unnamed Lady of the Castle.

A Story About the Story

I received a booking to tell a seasonal story one Friday in December. In the middle of the Tuesday night prior to the event, I entered a dream state, spontaneously telling myself the seasonal story of 'Sir Gawain and the Green Knight'. I rose early on Wednesday morning and wrote the story I had been telling myself in the night. The original story is of immense length, and I only had 20 minutes to tell it in. On Thursday I rehearsed.

On Friday, I told the story to the Business Women's Luncheon Club, in the French Dining Room, of the once infamous Cliveden Hotel, the first man to address this august body.

I took 30 minutes of the 20 minutes I had been given to speak. No one complained or walked out. Afterwards, a businesswoman approached me and said how much she had enjoyed listening to the story. I told her how the story had written itself in the middle of Tuesday night. She nodded sagely and said, "So, the story was channelled."

Synopsis

On the winter solstice, Sir Gawain accepts a challenge from a green knight to exchange blow for blow. Sir Gawain strikes the first blow and the green knight's head rolls away, only for the beheaded body to pick it up and ride away. In a 12 month, it is the green knight's turn. Sir Gawain rides north and is welcomed like a brother by the lord of a moated castle, close by the green knight's green chapel. Sir Gawain is enchanted by the lady of the castle. Each day, while her lord is in the field, the lady enjoys her flirtatious dalliance with Gawain in his elegant chamber, pressing her suit with wooing glances and sensual skirmishes, whilst he struggles to maintain his honour, parrying her fond forays with courtly grace. Finally, at the green chapel, he faces the green knight, and there arrives—in pantomime terms—The Reveal: will Gawain lose his head?

The Story

The Green Knight

It was the winter solstice at Camelot. King Arthur and Queen Guinevere led the revels. The great hall rang with the laughter of fair, feisty women sporting tall pointed hats and gowns of surpassing décolleté, and lusty knights, all of them quaffing hot spiced ale and mulled wine. The festive board groaned beneath a sumptuous fare of roast wild boar, whole swans, game pie, sucking pigs, a surfeit of lampreys, whole baked salmon, sweetmeats, gooseberry tarts, flagons of custard, …

As was his custom, King Arthur forbade the feasting to commence save first some fine test of skill or wondrous tale of derring-do. As he looked around for such as these, there came a wonder—crashing through the door with a mighty bellow, a warrior of giant size on a massive charger, clutching a gargantuan axe in a mailed fist and bearing a holly branch in his other hand. He galloped into the hall, the horse's hooves clattering on the paving stones, scattering sparks.

But the greatest wonder was that the knight was green. Green were his crown of curly locks, his face, his hood and cloak, his tunic and hose, and his boots and spurs. Likewise, his horse was green from forelock to fetlocks, from mane to tail, saddle, bit, and bridle.

Drawing his horse to a standstill, the Green Knight bellowed,

"Who is master here? I would speak with him." The king replied,

"Sir knight, welcome, I bid you dismount and share our feast and say your business here."

The Green Knight spoke again,

"I cannot tarry. As this holly bough bears witness, I come in peace, simply for seasonal sport." Gazing around, he went on, "I wonder which of these puny knights, these beardless boys, is willing to trade me blow for blow, wielding my axe? Let him leap forth and grasp it, and smite me where I stand. And here's the bargain, this day twelvemonth hence I get to return the blow. Who'll take my challenge?"

Incensed and red of face, the king leapt up, stretching out his hand for the axe, but Sir Gawain reached it first,

"Nay, sire, grant me this chance to prove my valour. I accept the challenge."

The Green Knight knelt, lifted his green locks over the crown of his head, and stretched out his neck. Sir Gawain hefted high the mighty axe, then whipped it down, severing bone and sinew in a single strike, sparking and splitting the stone. The green head rolled away, leaving a trail of green blood as it was kicked like a ball from foot to foot. There was utter shock and silence in the hall.

Then, slowly, the bloody corpse raised itself to its feet and walked stiffly to where its head lay, its green eyes open and bright. He lifted the head by its green locks, its eyes swivelling round to leer at Guinevere. The Green Knight mounted his great charger, holding the head aloft, and the green lips began to move,

"I am the Knight of the Green Chapel in the Northern waste. This day twelvemonth, Gawain, be there. I shall return the blow." Spurring his charger, with a clatter of hooves, the Green Knight was gone.

The Lady of the Castle

With the approach of the next Winter Solstice, Sir Gawain mounted his horse and left Camelot for the Northern waste to search out the Green Chapel. He drew near to northern Wales, close by the Isle of Anglesey, rode over shallow water near the sea, and wandered o'er the wilderness of Wirral where few respected God or mortal with goodwill. He was drenched by winter rain and sleet. He stumbled into deep snowdrifts. He slept night after night on the frozen ground.

Finally, he came to a moated castle, its painted pinnacles glistening in the early morning light. The lord of the castle welcomed him like a brother. The lord was red-haired, red-bearded, tall and tough as a tree with a trunk to match, with a massive appetite for stories and laughter. He led Sir Gawain to a chamber hung with rich tapestries. There was a bed of soft down with quilted coverlets curtained in silk brocade.

At dinner, Sir Gawain met the lady of the castle. As their eyes met, 'twas like for him a peal of festive bells.

Red was her robe, and cluster of clear pearls
Gleamed in her head-dress; breast and throat were bare,
Whiter than snow which lies on winter hills,
Her eyes a twinkle, her manner debonair,
And never had he seen a face so fair.

By her side was an ancient crone swathed in musty veils and dark raiment, whom Sir Gawain barely noticed in the light of the lady's face. After dinner they retired to the hall where the lord and lady entertained Sir Gawain with stories and revelry, carolling and carousing, laughter and leaping dance.

Sir Gawain told of his dire quest to meet the Green Knight just three days hence.

"Why, the Green Chapel is barely two miles distance. Here you can rest and nourish yourself. For three days whilst you rest I shall go a-hunting. My wife shall keep you company at home. So, let us make a bargain. All I win in the chase is yours. Whatever you win is mine." They raised their mugs of ale to swear their oath.

Courtly Dalliance, One Kiss

The lord arose at cockcrow and took the field. Meanwhile, Sir Gawain lazed in his bed of down, beneath the coverlets, with silk curtains drawn. There was a soft click as the door quietly opened. Soft footfalls crossed the floor. The lady slid the curtain aside, laughter quivering on her lips,

"Why, sire, I find the sentry sleeping at his post. Perchance, I shall bind him to his bed." So saying, she sat on the bed and leant towards him.

"Madam, I am your prisoner. I pray you, release me. Let me rise and dress." She shook her head,

"Perhaps I shall let you rise. But dress? By no means, not whilst I have the bravest knight in the land at my behest, with my liege lord far away in the field. I offer you my lips, my love, my treasure. Why, I see the sentry has risen and stands at his post."

"Madam, madam, for honour's sake, alas, I must refuse. You have chosen a better lord. Yet, I will pledge to serve you as your liegeman."

And so, with wooing glances, subtle taunts and amorous advances, she toyed with him. Whilst he parried each foray with courtly grace and deftly turned her gibes to harmless jest, until the morning passed most pleasantly away.

"Surely," she said at last, "after so long a sojourn, the gentle knight might crave at least a kiss before we part."

"Madam, 'tis my courtly duty to obey." She clasped him in her arms, kissed him, and withdrew.

That evening in the hall, the lord heaped up his winnings for the day, wild boar, their blood running over the flagstones,

"All for you, sire, this was our bargain." Sir Gawain clasped him by the shoulder,

"My winnings, lord, a fair exchange, one kiss."

"Why," said the lord, "what delight. How came you by this?"

"Ah!" replied Sir Gawain, "That was no part of our bargain. I will not say." So, jesting, they went in to dine.

Courtly Dalliance, Two Kisses

The next day the lord arose at cockcrow and took the field. Meanwhile, Sir Gawain lazed in his bed of down, beneath the coverlets, with silk curtains drawn. And there the lady tiptoed to him, withdrew the curtains, and breathed his name.

So, as before, they entered into courtly dalliance, the amorous word, the wooing glance, parrying fond forays with courtly grace. Until,

"My liege lord is far away in the chase. This moment he scents a deer, its soft nose warm and moist, hidden in a bush. Why should those who lie abed be denied such thrilling sport."

"Madam, madam, I would fain cast away my honour and virtue to enter such a chase. Yet, I will not, I will not for all that."

"Why, sire, have you forgot even what I taught you but yester-morn of courtliness and kissing?" And with that, she stole two kisses and was gone.

That evening, the lord displayed his winnings, a soft-nosed deer with a red gash in its side.

"For you, sire, as we agreed." Sir Gawain clasped him by the neck,

"My winnings, lord, two kisses." "Why," said the lord, "two kisses. Such increase in your trade. How came you by such fortune?"

"Ah!" replied Sir Gawain, "I will not say." So, laughing, they went in to dine.

Courtly Dalliance, Three Kisses, Green Girdle

The next day the lord arose at cockcrow and took the field. Meanwhile, Sir Gawain lazed in his bed of down, beneath the coverlets, with silk curtains drawn. The lady came with purpose fell, threw back the blinds and curtains, and let the winter sun stream in.

She stood before him, her finest red wrap trailing to the ground, her arms akimbo, diamonds at her throat and clustered in her hair, her back and bosom bare.

"For shame, for shame, that here you lie and snore when the morning beams so bright, and with our time so short for courtly love? Arise, arise!"

She bounced onto the bed, her wrap slipping from her shoulders, and stooping low she gave him one kiss. One kiss, and all the bliss of blossom time was his. Hard the lady pressed her loving charms,

"My liege lord is far away in the field. This moment he is facing a she-wolf, whose lascivious, slavering jaws yearn to embrace his living flesh. Why should those who lie abed be denied such perilous sport."

Sir Gawain cried in anguish,

"Heaven forefend I should deceive my noble host, and yet, I love thee with all my heart and soul." The lady kissed him deeply, thrice, then drawing back unfurled from round her narrow waist a silken girdle, green, enriched with stones of jade and emerald and green pearls.

"T'is a talisman of magic worth, so potent it will shield you from any blade. Wear it beneath your mantle when you meet the Green Knight. But promise, lest I be chastised, breath no word to my lord."

That evening in the hall, Sir Gawain spoke,

"This night let me be first to pay." Grasping the lord by the neck he delivered three kisses.

"Three kisses!" laughed the lord, "Rich merchandise, a bounty I shall treasure. And the price you paid?"

"That's no part of our bargain. My payment's made."

"Then here is mine," said the lord. He displayed his winnings for the day, "A ferocious she-wolf, cut down like a dog, a poor return for a gift of priceless worth, three precious kisses." Of the green girdle, Sir Gawain spoke no word.

"It is enough," he said and, embarrassed, turned away.

The Green Chapel

A reluctant dawn broke on a Winter Solstice joyless, bitter and bleak. Sir Gawain bid farewell to his host and rode slowly towards the Green Chapel, in a narrow sheer-sided valley, sunless and dank, with rank grasses and scrubby trees, where no birds sang. The green bejewelled girdle was bound about his waist in hope it might shield him from hurt.

As he approached the Green Chapel and dismounted, he heard the whirring of the grindstone and the whining of the Green Knight's axe being sharpened to a fine edge. Then the Green Knight appeared, hefting his axe, his great bulk blotting out what little light there was in the sunless valley.

"Twelvemonth past you lopped off my head. Now, I shall return the kindness," said the Green Knight.

"I am not afraid," replied Sir Gawain.

"Then ready yourself to receive the blow."

Sir Gawain knelt and stretched out his neck. As he heard the whistle of the falling axe, he flinched. At the last moment, the giant stopped the axe in mid-air, hovering over Gawain's neck.

"You are not Gawain, the courageous knight who fears no foe, if you flinch at the whistle of the blade. At Camelot, I never shied away."

"Alas," replied Sir Gawain, "my head when it falls will never be restored to my shoulders. I shall not flinch again. Strike!"

The Green Knight whirled the axe around his head for speed, then with a roar he brought it down, side-slipping at the last moment and plunging the blade into the earth.

"Now you have found your nerve, I shall strike all the harder," he said.

"I'm weary of your bullying," replied Sir Gawain, "Let's have no more delay."

"Then take your pay."

The giant spat on his hands and again hefted the great axe, raised it high and brought it down with all his power and strength. No power on earth could save Sir Gawain now. The axe hurtled towards his bared neck, so guided by the Green Knight it gave Sir Gawain's neck the smallest graze, three drops of his bright blood staining the snow.

Unbelieving, Sir Gawain leapt to his feet, snatched up his sword and stood at guard,

"You've had your blow. You shall have no other. I have kept the covenant we made at Camelot. Now, I'm ready to pit my strength and skill at arms against yours."

The Green Knight leant on his axe,

"I'll strike no more. You have been true to the covenant we made. I shall explain. The first and second strikes were deliberate feints, for you honoured your pledges given to the lord, one kiss, two kisses, from the lady of the castle. In return for the she-wolf you gave three kisses more, yet you paid the lord falsely, for you held back the green girdle, and for this I grazed your skin. Yet, I forgive you, for you are a true knight; you failed the final test not out of desire for riches or pleasures of the flesh but simply for loving your life. Moreover, I too have held something back—the lady is my wife."

"Your wife!" cried Sir Gawain, mortified with shame and disgrace, "Alas, I have betrayed the laws of chivalry and my honour as a knight."

"Not so," laughed the Green Knight, "my wife was keen to learn the lore and language of courtly love through practice with one well versed in those arts. Moreover, I have been under an enchantment by the old hag to whom you paid so little heed, none other than Morgan le Faye, who sought to bring dishonour upon Camelot's finest and most honourable knight. So, now your honour is intact and the spell is broke."

Gawain Has Lost His Head

Returning to Camelot, Sir Gawain truthfully told his tale, showing the scar the axe had made and displaying the green girdle. Yet, he was racked with grief, chagrin, and shame for the tarnish on his name, though others made fun of him, parading their own green girdles.

Yet, Sir Gawain's heart still dwelt with the lady, for the courtly knight had lost his head to her.

Red was her robe, and cluster of clear pearls
Gleamed in her head-dress; breast and throat were bare,
Whiter than snow which lies on winter hills,
Her eyes a twinkle, her manner debonair,
And never had he seen a face so fair.

In bitter shame and loss and grief, Sir Gawain hung his head and would ne'er be comforted.

Sources

Sir Gawain and the Green Knight is a long anonymous poem, one of the masterpieces of English literature, a late 14th-century chivalric romance in Middle English. The poem only survives in a single manuscript at the British Library.

I acknowledge the author of that beautiful poetic version of *Sir Gawain and the Green Knight* from which I have quoted the poem, but whose name I have failed to discover.

I acknowledge Annette Armstrong, whose free translation of *Gawain & The Green Knight* (October 2003) provided invaluable source material and some phraseology.

Reflections

Your Psychological Reflection

Gawain seizes hold of the Green Knight's challenge to prove his valour. He endures severe privations on his journey north, not least the godless wilderness of Wirral (Godly citizens of Wirral, sorry to offend!). Meeting the lady of the castle is like a peal of festive bells for him; he fancies her. So, resisting her charms was a taxing trial of honour. Then, instead of acceding to her demands and enjoying the pleasure, he merely succumbs to her silken green girdle. He can be forgiven the flinch; he was pretty courageous kneeling for the axe. Finally, he is racked with grief, chagrin, and shame for the tarnish on his name. Could this be a Soul Crisis?

When you gaze beneath the surface of this tale with your therapist's eyes, what do you discern? How surprised are you by the power relationship between the characters? Who holds the power? How well versed really is Sir Gawain in the art of courtly love? Has he proved his valour?

Is this really a tale of courtly love or a dark tale of intrigue, deceit, and control?

What is the reason for Gawain being racked with such grief, chagrin, and shame? Loss of the lady? Feeling inadequate as a courtly lover? Losing his honour by succumbing to the lure of the lady's silken green girdle? All of these reasons? Something else?

I invite you to track the dynamic portrayal of Gawain's Soul through the story.

Courtly Love Then and Now

In medieval times, a chivalric knight would pledge his courtly love and devotion to a lady, even a married lady; knight and lady would be free to speak openly about love and romance, sharing poems and songs of love, alluding to sexual pleasures without going beyond the bounds of what was considered propriety.

In recent times, sex therapist David Schnarch (*Constructing the Sexual Crucible,* 1991), in his reflections about "sex beyond the orgasmic threshold," writes, "We are a society in which the goal of sexuality is orgasms. … Yet the human body is capable of ecstatic phenomenological experiences beyond orgasm for which there is no known physiological counterpart."

David Schnarch asks questions that smack of courtly love, "Does orgasm represent the limits of human sexual experience? Is there some aspect of subjective intensity in sexual experience that might be independent of the physiological event of orgasm? If so, why are many people seemingly unaware of this?" He maintains, "Peak transcendent experience lies at the further reaches of human sexual potential."

{Wow!}

My Psychological Reflection

David Schnarch asks, "Is there some aspect of subjective intensity in sexual experience that might be independent of the physiological event of orgasm?" It seems there was courtly love in medieval times, so why not today? Surely, two people can enter a deep, loving, trusting, creative, intimate union that falls short of coitus. To my mind, such courtly love is possible between people in the transpersonal phase, who may suffer the urge to merge whilst remaining separate.

Falling in love or feeling strong sexual attraction outside of a committed relationship is not uncommon, and the urge to merge is difficult to resist, variously resulting in deception, turmoil, anger, and perhaps most of all shame. I know situations where having an affair is actually a symptom of an unacknowledged spiritual crisis prompting a relationship crisis, and in a psychotherapeutic context it is the spiritual crisis that calls to be addressed.

The realisation of courtly love emerging between two people in the transpersonal phase—whether at a time of spiritual crisis or not—means each party acknowledging and suffering the urge to merge. Everything has a meaning, so allowing and embracing the emotional pain of the urge to merge, enables meaning to be revealed, thereby deepening the relationship. Courtly love emerging without merging is the key to a 'subjective intensity in sexual experience' that is open and untainted by shame.

What of Sir Gawain? After three days of courtly dalliance, with the lady pressing her loving charms, he finally succumbs, if only to the lady's silken green girdle. This is the meaning I take from the story, succumbing destroys courtly love and leaves shame in its wake.

Pearl of Wisdom

> *There is a well-known bawdy campfire tale that I have heard told many times, 'The Woman Who Had Two'. I have taken this tale and raised it to another level, and frankly I love my version.*
>
> *After telling this tale, a woman listener looked at me with a frown and asked, "Two what?"*

A story can state an existential dilemma briefly and pointedly,
in a way which resonates with the listener's own inner conflicts,
so they can imagine themselves healed and being whole.

Synopsis

A king with an inflated belief in his own sexual prowess and with bizarre and unimaginable sexual fantasies seeks to select a wife with whom to fulfil his desires. It is of course the wife who selects him, as women do. She is more than he bargained for. She is intent on fulfilling his—and her own—deepest yearnings.

The Story

Once there was a woman who lived with her mother. She was as beautiful as her mother was poor. The woman was tall and voluptuous. She had the fine looks of a noble Egyptian. Her nose was exquisite. Her hair was a dark amber, full and flowing. Her eyes were at once dark and bright. And she had such a soft, dark down on her as would drive a man to distraction.

Her only possession of any worth was a sandalwood box which had been in her family for generations. It was intricately carved, with a fine network of tiny holes worked into the lid.

Now, the king of that country was tall and strong, and one day he decided it was time he took a wife to be his queen, to be his life companion, and to assist him with the affairs of state. Thinking himself a lusty fellow, he decided he would only marry a woman who had two. So, he put out a proclamation throughout the land:

> *Hear ye, hear ye! The king announces that he wishes to marry and will receive applications to be queen from any woman who has two.*

Thousands of young women, and some not so young, besieged the palace, eager to be queen. Each one was directed to the office of the Grand Vizier, whose job it was to study their applications and to scrutinise their credentials. The Grand Vizier was diligent in his work. He was willing to apply himself for long hours each day. He enjoyed his work. But he found no applicant with the necessary qualifications to be queen.

The woman's mother, like many mothers throughout the land, urged her daughter to attend the palace and try her luck, but the woman said,

"No! I will wait." And the more the poor woman urged her daughter to attend the palace the more she refused,

"No! I will wait."

The flow of applicants dwindled from thousands to hundreds to dozens to just a trickle each day, until the day when there was no applicant at all. The king was disappointed and frustrated. On the following day, the woman put on her finest raiment, drew a veil over her face, took the sandalwood box, and made her way to the palace, where she was directed to the office of the Grand Vizier.

"No!" she said, "I'm not going to present myself to some Grand Voyeur. I will only deal directly with the king."

Well, as the sole remaining applicant they could hardly refuse, and so she was brought before the king.

"You have the necessary qualifications?" asked the king.

"I do," she replied.

"So, show me," he said.

"Certainly not," she replied, "What sort of women do you think I am. Not until you have married with me."

"Well," said the king, "at least remove your veil and let me see your face."

So, she removed her veil and he gazed in delight upon her fine looks, as of a noble Egyptian, her exquisite nose, her hair a dark amber, full and flowing, and her eyes at once dark and bright. And the soft, dark down of her drove him to distraction. So, the Grand Vizier was called as witness, and they made their vows to be true to one another and to make the journey of love together until their time shall pass away.

Then they were escorted to the bedchamber prepared for a queen, should she be found. When they were alone, the king kissed her gently and said,

"Now, show me."

And so, she unveiled herself to him. She had such a voluptuous beauty on her as was renowned for centuries, and even a thousand years later the singers of the Song of Songs, the Sacred Marriage, recalled her as the model for their bride:

"Behold, thou art fair, my love, behold thou art surpassing fair.
Thy nose is as the Tower of Lebanon that looketh toward Damascus,
And the smell of thy nose is like apples.
Thy breasts are like twin fawns feasting upon lilies.
Thy stature is like unto a palm tree,
And thy breasts to clusters of grapes.
Thy belly is like to an heap of wheat set about with lilies.
Verily, the joy of thee is as a pure translucent pearl in a setting of dark amber.

Yea, the joy of thee is as a song bird, so feathery and soft and warm and pulsing
with life beneath the bridegroom's hand."

"But," said the king huffily, "you only have one. You promised me two, but you have only one."

She laughed, deep and sultry,

"I don't wear them both at once. We can only use one at a time. I keep the spare in this little sandalwood box."

And she showed him the sandalwood box, so intricately carved with its network of tiny holes worked into the lid.

By now the royal sceptre was risen keen as a sickle at harvest. This was no time to quibble over contracts. And so, they entered into one another and loved one another in every imaginable way and every unimaginable way and the months passed in joy.

Now, the queen had a fine bedchamber, with a great window looking to the south, and each day she put out crumbs and tiny sweetmeats for the birds, so that they came to know and trust her and became her friends.

One day, the king came to her, as she always knew he would, to tell her he must make a long journey to a distant land. And he asked, rather shyly for a great king, as he was to be away for some time, if he might take the spare.

"Why, of course, my love," said the queen, "that way I can journey with you. I will bring it to you as you depart."

And so, when the birds came to visit her windowsill, she took a young wren gently in her hands, carefully placed it in the sandalwood box, so intricately carved with its network of tiny holes worked into the lid, along with water and sweetmeats.

She brought the sandalwood box with its precious contents to the king.

"Take good care of it," she said to him, "for it would be a tragedy if our only spare were to be lost."

After journeying for several days, the king came to an arbour of cherry trees all in blossom, where a bank of soft grass, warm in the sun, sloped down to a gentle stream arched by sweet willow. He removed his clothing, lay down on the warm grass, and took, into his hand, the sandalwood box.

As he slipped his hand inside the box and felt what was within, so feathery and soft and warm and pulsing with life beneath his hand, the royal sceptre rose keen as a sickle at harvest. He opened the box, and joyful for its release the young wren flew up and away and was gone. The king was mortified that in his passion he had lost the only spare beyond hope of retrieval. After that his journey was long and bitter.

In the absence of the king, the queen ruled the land with patience, good sense, and sharp attention. Except, her ministers noticed, from time to time she would muse a space and a secret smile would flit across her lips, as she conducted the affairs of state.

The day came when the watchmen called that the king was in sight. The queen retired to her bedchamber, where the king joined her immediately upon his arrival.

"A terrible thing has happened," he blurted out, "I have lost the spare."

He fell to his knees, his head drooping in despair.

"Well, my love," she said, as she took him by the hand and raised him up, "that is indeed a terrible thing, but we shall just have to make the best use we can of the one which remains."

And so, they entered into one another afresh. They stroked and caressed one another with fragrant oils. They shared their feelings and felt for one another. They told each other stories and poems and sang songs. And they argued and fought and struggled together. They reflected together in simple contemplation, quietness and peace. They loved one another in every imaginable way and every unimaginable way, and laughed and laughed together, for there is no laughter so glorious as the laughter of the bedchamber.

And slowly, and in due time, as his manhood grew, the king came to realise how his wife, the queen, had had two all along, how she still had two, of the body and of the soul. And so, they ruled the land with majesty and power, and lived and journeyed one with the other, in that mysterious conjoining of difference which is the very soul of conjugal love. Until their time shall pass away.

Source

Loosely based on the popular campfire tale *The Woman Who Had Two*. If you know the origin of this well-told tale, please, let me know.

Reflections

Egalitarian Reflection

Like many insightful folk tales, *Pearl of Wisdom* is about the redemption of man by woman. Of equal moment, the story is about a woman who can both exercise her power in a man's world and fulfil her role in deepening the intimate relationship with her lover in every delectable sense.

Your Psychological Reflection

Enjoy the wit, <u>will</u>, and wise eroticism of this exquisite, alluring woman. I wish you joy in appraising her <u>Sexuality</u> and <u>Portrayal of Soul</u>. The king as well, of course.

My Psychological Reflection

Nathan Schwartz-Salant (1998) writes about relationships, "All people need a partner in the effort to individuate if this integrative path is to include love, aggression, and bodily life, along with a spiritual focus of values and goals. Rarely, if ever, can a person enter the path of creating and transforming a self without the fire and challenge of an ongoing relationship."

A couple in the pre-personal, ego-building phase of the Journey of Soulmaking carry into the relationship their differing 'ways of being', the values, beliefs, attitudes, and aspirations they assimilated as they grew up, bringing the likelihood of conflict. A couple in the personal self phase is likely to be equally fraught when each seeks to assert their own opinions. Being in different phases, for example, one being submissive and the other assertive, may be a recipe for avoiding conflict at the cost of discontent and stagnation.

What I take from the Schwartz-Salant quotation is that couple therapy can be an alchemical crucible within which to refine the gold of intimacy Soul-to-Soul, and our role as therapist is to serve as a catalyst, aiding this nascent transmutation of Soul. What this means for me is that couple therapy is not about applying sticking plasters but about the long-term fire and challenge of mutual psychological growth.

I sometimes encounter couple clients in different phases, as in the story. The king is caught in grandiosity and stuck in a bizarre conviction about what it means to be his queen. Unphased by her inauspicious situation, knowing her worth, and in possession of her precious sandalwood box, the woman patiently plans her future, sharpens her wits, and selects her moment when she can choose the king. Then, with patience, wit, good sense, and sharp attention, she gently leads him into that mysterious conjoining of difference which is the very soul of transpersonal love. It is a joy and privilege to work with such as these in the therapy room.

Note

1 The Convent of the Sacred Heart of Mary is actually a Grade II Listed Building in Upminster, London, maintained by Historic England, https://historicengland.org.uk/listing/the-list/list-entry/1387179?section=official-list-entry.

Bibliography

Armstrong, Annette (October 2003) *Gawain & The Green Knight*, free translation.

Arnold, Matthew (1867) *Dover Beach and Other Poems.*

Berry, A. J. (1912) *The Story of Preston*, Sir Isaac Pitman & Sons.

Boccaccio, Giovanni (ca. 1353) *The Decameron.*

Clarke, Peter (Written, 1715), Paton, Henry M. A. (Ed., 1893) *'A Journall of Severall Occurrences from 2nd November 1715, in the Insurrection (began in Scotland) and Concluded at Preston in Lancashire, on November 14, MDCCXV'*, kept by Peter Clarke, being Part I of *'Papers About the Rebellions of 1715 and 1745, Edited from the Original Manuscripts, with Introduction and Notes'*, Henry Paton M. A., Printed at the University Press by T. and A. Constable for the Scottish History Society.

England, David and Bilbé, Tina (2013) *Berkshire Folk Tales*, The History Press.

Fishwick, Henry and Ditchfield, P. H. (Eds) (1909) *Memorials of old Lancashire (Volumes I and II)*, Bemrose & Sons.

Gray, Rosemary (Ed.) (c1986) *The Book of Wargrave*, Wargrave Local History Society.
Hird, Frank (1912) *Lancashire Stories, Volumes I & II, Containing All that Appeals to the Heart and the Imagination in the Lancashire of Today and of Many Yesterdays*, T C and E C Jack.
Schnarch, David M. (1991) *Constructing the Sexual Crucible*. W. W. Norton.
Wikipedia, *Eleusinian Mysteries*. https://en.wikipedia.org/wiki/Baubo

Beastly Tales Room

From earliest times, beasts have burrowed into the souls of human beings, nesting, nestling, and roosting until emerging in ancient tales as shape-shifting creatures, creatures of romance, creatures of fear and fun, creatures of wonder, creatures of nightmare—a shadow of the real-life horror spewing from the tormented mind of man.

I had doubts about including this Room in a collection of traditional tales set within a psychological context. However, to my surprise, as I worked on the Room, I realised that three of the tales could have been included in the Transpersonal Tales Room, whilst some tales touch upon the suffering of women at the hands of men. There remains just one I included because I like it and because it's fun.

Not all beasts are beastly, though the 'Unsworth Dragon' certainly is, so keep him well away from your wives and daughters. The 'Great Hairy Toe' was once attached to a really beastly beast, though he does have an affectionate side. As does the worm in 'King Gaarge and the Dragon', until the beastly King Gaarge did for him anyway. The shape-shifting creatures in 'Lady Sybil and the Milk White Doe' are beast-like rather than beastly. In 'The Witches Of Windsor' it's people who are beastly.

DOI: 10.4324/9781003712329-8

The Unsworth Dragon

> *Beware! The Unsworth Dragon is an exceptionally bloodthirsty beast, with, alas, a particular appetite for women.*
>
> *Discussing stories of English dragons, Harland & Wilkinson tell us, "There is a singular circumstance connected with these dragon stories. It is that of the frequent use of sacred and mystic numbers in the narratives, and this supports the conjecture that they are allegorical in their nature." Harland & Wilkinson refer to the Dragon of Wantley with its seven heads and twice seven eyes eating up three children. In 'The Unsworth dragon', I have remained faithful to this singular circumstance and used sacred and mystic numbers throughout.*

Let the story tell the story.
The story enables the listener to generate a new way of experiencing themselves, which at the outset is unknown.

Synopsis

For many generations, a fierce and terrible dragon has ravaged the surrounding country from its lair near Unsworth. The dragon has burst from the forest again, defying the prowess of sundry brave heroes to slay it. However, Thomas Unsworth, perceiving that the dragon's scaly hide is invulnerable to bullets, loads his dagger into his petronel. He rouses the monster's ire with a feigned attack. He shoots the dragon in the throat when it raises its head. The dagger pierces the throat's soft skin. Thomas ends the cycle.

Later, an oak table is made with carved images, one of them the figure of a worm with the face of a man. Who can he be?

The Story

Hund was one of the hound clan, the Hundingas. With a lean, powerful stature, a swarthy complexion, eyes of pitch, sunken and suspicious, a long nose and heavy jowls, and a perpetually mournful visage, he looked half hound himself. Fiercely independent, Hund had departed from the main settlement at Bury with a small group of followers and some sheep and cattle to form his own Hund's Settlement, a day's journey to the south.

They had toiled from sunrise to sunset, clearing the ground for the settlement and for pasture and crops, then tilling the soil, planting and harvesting their wheat, barley and rye, and husbanding their animals. There had been couplings between man and woman, and children added to their community. Hund's woman had given him one child, a boy of seven years.

Thus, they had followed the cycle of the seasons, developing their settlement, for seven years. One day towards dusk a stranger arrived at the settlement, a woman of exquisite beauty. She wore a belted gown with tight sleeves to the wrist and an outer garment with shorter, looser sleeves, both ankle length, made of wool of the finest quality. To show her freedom, her copper-coloured hair was unbound and uncovered, falling to her shoulders, and she carried a long dagger at her belt.

The woman asked to stay for three nights and was quickly made welcome. She listened attentively to the women, deftly fended off the attentions of the men, and laughed and played with the children, especially making friends with Hund's son and winning his confidence.

The woman was careful always to remain in the shade, for she cast no shadow.

On the third day, in the gathering dusk, the woman drew Hund's son aside to a quiet place at the edge of the settlement. She took from her loose robe a bright shiny apple impaled upon her dagger's tip and handed it to the boy with a gentle smile. The boy took the apple with shining eyes, for apples were out of season. He ate with relish, core and all, as the woman watched. For a moment her smile turned to malevolent glee, her copper hair faded to ash, and her face collapsed into a cadaverous mask, then she was gone.

At the core of the apple was a tiny worm. It squirmed its way through the boy's body to the root of his spine, where it lay dormant for five times seven years. By that time Hund's son had taken over from Hund as chief of the settlement. He had Hund's hound-like countenance. He had a young son. One day the worm awoke and began to wriggle its way up Hund's son's spinal column, causing him immense torment.

In agony, Hund's son rushed from the settlement into the nearby forest. There, the worm worked its will on his sinews, bones and flesh, relentlessly tearing, turning, twisting, stretching, an orgasmic ecstasy of pain, until man became worm.

Hund's son might soon have been missed had calamity not overtaken the settlement. A dragon burst out of the forest and began at once to devour the sheep.

{A quick reminder, English dragons are giant worms.}

A young shepherd rushed forward to protect his flock, waving his crook. The serpent opened his great maw and brought it down over the boy's head and shoulders. The other shepherds saw his legs flailing as he was sucked into the worm's capacious crop.

The people poured out of the settlement with spears and axes to fight and kill the dragon, but these weapons were useless against his impenetrable hide. Many perished in the skirmish, slithering down into the creature's commodious crop.

Once the worm's desire for flesh was satisfied, he withdrew into the forest, only to re-emerge the next day, and the next. For seven weeks of seven long days the dragon ravaged the land for miles around, gorging on the people as they tended their crops and animals.

The dragon had a partiality for females. However vigilant a woman might be, the worm had a way of coming upon her unawares, burrowing through the earth and bursting out behind her. A moment too late, she would turn to be transfixed by recognition before the great maw gulped her into its gullet: the dragon bore the familial hound-face of Hund's son.

One woman, or more than one, was able to flee. The serpent caught her with his tail and gathered her in his coils. He crushed her till her bones cracked, then lifting her aloft he let go. She fell, her eyes wide with terror, screaming and flailing, head-first down the gaping gullet of Hund's son.

From the worm's crop radiated the hot stench of blood and decaying flesh, the acrid reek of lost wives and daughters drifting across the fields and settlements.

After seven weeks, Hund's son staggered back into the settlement, naked and confused, with no notion of his whereabouts these long weeks.

Memory of the dragon evoked such horror it was rarely spoken of, and as one generation succeeded another the memory faded.

After twice seven generations, Hund's successor, also called Hund, was smitten by a strange malady making him cringe with excruciating pain; like an army of ants, he screamed, crawling beneath his skin. In agony, he rushed from the settlement into the forest. The worm had returned.

For seven weeks of seven long days the dragon decimated the womenfolk all around, sucking them into his crop in the very moment they recognised the familial face of Hund, grinding them in his gizzard. The pungent odour of death from the worm's crop reached across the landscape. After that time, Hund returned to the settlement, naked and befuddled.

After twice seven generations, the dragon returned, devastating the hamlet, then again after a further twice seven generations…

I am Thomas Unsworth. I am a young man living in the village of Unsworth. This is now my story.

I become anxious about my father, Squire Thomas, who complained of agonising pain, like fiends with sharp fangs feasting upon his vitals. Then, abruptly he disappeared. As I wondered what had happened to him, I heard a commotion in the village. I rushed out to find the villagers scurrying around in terror of a fierce dragon which had just emerged from the forest and was gobbling up the women working in the fields before they could flee.

Several knights with manors nearby donned their armour, took their lances and swords, and rode out fearlessly to face the dragon. Alas, swords and lances glanced uselessly off the worm's tough coils. The dragon swallowed the knights whole and shat out their armour. Some knights took up their harquebuses and petronels and fired at the dragon. It was futile. Even a sustained harquebusade failed to deter the beast from his feasting.

{Harquebus, harquebusade, petronel, serpentine trigger, such gloriously obsolete words for antique long firearms are a joy to employ. The petronel has a serpent-shaped trigger to apply a smouldering rope match to the flash pan, boom!}

Unsworth Dragon

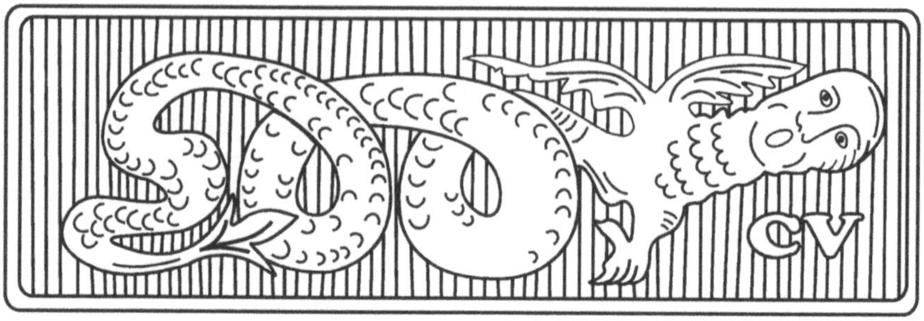

Figure 6.1 The Unsworth Dragon Illustrator Joanne Lowes.

Seeing the failure of the fusillade and fearing my father had been taken by the dragon, I devised a plan. I cleaned and primed my father's petronel. I loaded his long dagger into the firearm's barrel. I lit the slow-burn rope match and clamped it onto the serpentine trigger beside the flash pan. I donned my father's old black armour and belted on his sword.

Now, thus equipped and attired, I mount my father's faithful charger—which has seen many a tourney, though none like this—click my lance into its rest, and with the petronel held firmly against my chest I canter out, like St George *{or King Gaarge}* to fight the dragon.

I find the worm with the legs of three children slipping through his jaws. Horrified, I raise my lance. I charge the dread creature at full tilt, knowing the lance will be of no avail save to provide a diversion. At the last moment I drop the lance, just as the dragon lowers his head and opens his fetid, suffocating, slavering maw. With my right hand now free, I pull the serpentine trigger to ignite the priming powder, bellowing, "Set a serpent to slay a serpent."

In this exultant moment, as the dagger blasts from the barrel, fatally tearing a jagged hole in the dragon's throat, I look up into my father's beloved face.

Note

Mortified at being the cause of his father's death, notwithstanding the dread circumstances, Thomas Unsworth had a carved oak table made for him, in memory of his father and of the events surrounding his death.[1]

Sources

Harland, John and Wilkinson, T. T. (1873), p. 63; Hird, Frank (1912), Volume I p. 104.

First published in Lancashire Folk Tales (Jennie Bailey and David England, 2014).

Reflections

Your Psychological Reflection

I invite you to take Harland & Wilkinson's suggestion that dragon stories are allegorical in their nature and reflect on what *The Unsworth Dragon* allegory might be. As a literary form, an allegory is a narrative in which characters, places, and events can be interpreted to represent a meaning, in this case, with psychological significance.

My Psychological and Egalitarian Reflection

A woman of shadows with dark intent gives an apple to a boy. The apple is out of right season and rotten to the core. The abusive injury, inflicted by the woman on the boy, dragonnades the family, generation after generation, like the ouroboros dragon chewing upon its own tail, each generation venting its rage and retribution on womankind. It's women who take the brunt.

An ouroboros dragon chewing upon its own tail is an apt metaphor for a family trapped in the maintaining cycle of an acquired mindset, an attitude of resentment and contempt towards women, often exhibited as: domestic abuse, gaslighting, coercive control, and predatory sexual conduct. The cycle is only broken when a son—or maybe a daughter—of the family attains a personal self, questions their acquired mindset, and asserts their own family choice.

King Gaarge and the Dragon

Suitable for older children

When you stand on White Horse Hill, above Dragon Hill, as I have done many times, gaze at the surrounding landscape; you can believe the dragon's great bulk scored those deep channels in the earth. I was there as part of a BBC Countryfile programme, set in Berkshire, to talk about Dragon Hill, and had my 75 seconds of fame.

This tale blends together two folk myths:

King Gaarge killed the dragon on Dragon Hill, and where its blood was spilt nothing will ever grow.

Dragon Hill is the burial mound of Uther Pendragon.

Then, another English dragon is added to the mix, 'The Laidly Worm of Spindleston Heugh', evidence that English dragons are really giant worms.

I am embarrassed to tell you, at the age of 5 I had the horrible, inexplicable experience of awakening one morning to find a large worm coming out of my behind. This worm has wormed its way into this story, coming out as an English dragon.

We sin against the imagination when we ask a story for its meaning.

Synopsis

Ethelinda, a milkmaid, is the narrator of this tale. She wakes one morning to find an earthworm on her pillow. She keeps it as a pet and it grows to be an English dragon, which she calls Draca. A local warrior chieftain dies and is buried under a mound by soldiers with all his gold. Dragons love gold and no sooner had the soldiers left than Draca took possession of the mound and its gold, and only let Ethelinda go near it. It's Draca's Dun now. The gold makes Draca ravenous. He eats mice at first and works up to sheep, then it's milkmaids he has an appetite for. The men say, "Something's got to be done about that Laidly Worm," and draw lots for a maiden a day for Draca's dinner with six pails of milk. One day, it's Ethelinda that's chosen and left for Draca's din. She's not happy. Draca's not happy. Then bumptious King Gaarge turns up. It's not a happy ending.

The Story

Everybody has a serpent inside, so they say, coiled at the base of the spine. I know it's true for me, because when I was six I woke one morning to find mine coiled on my pillow. It looked like a large earthworm, pinkish purple in colour. It seemed quite friendly for an earthworm, so we decided to keep it as a pet. That's my little sister Wynflaeth, which means beautiful and fair in our language, which she was, and me, Ethelinda, which means noble snake. My mother and father should never have called me that, or the tragedy which followed might never have happened.

We chopped up leftover vegetables to feed my worm, and it grew very quickly: it was 12 inches long in no time, so we called it Draca, which means dragon in our language, because English dragons are really big worms, not like those Welsh dragons I've heard of with wings and fiery breath.

Draca had no eyes or ears, so it couldn't see or hear us, yet it always sensed when someone was there, even whether it was either Wynflaeth or me. One day, Draca disappeared; there was just a round hole in the earth it must have made when it crawled off. Then it popped its head out of the soil and waved it about, like it was saying, "Pepo!" We loved to watch the way it stretched and contracted its body to slither along; we were amazed how quick it could go.

We spent a lot of our spare time with Draca, Wynflaeth and me, when we weren't herding the sheep or milking the cows or harvesting the crops. He loved it when I tickled the top of his head and waved his tail with delight. When he became big enough, Draca let us ride on his back as he rushed across the fields. He seemed to enjoy it as much as Wynflaeth and me.

Then something terrible happened. The land for miles and miles around was ruled by a warrior chieftain called Uther Pendragon. When he died they decided to bury him near us, just below our hill fort, which had been one of his favourite places, apparently. They built a great big burial mound, rocks of chalk covered by a thin layer of earth, and buried Uther in the middle of it along with all the golden treasure he'd got as Pendragon.

But that wasn't the terrible part. The terrible part was what happened to Draca. It seemed like he could smell the golden treasure. When the warriors arrived with Uther's body and his treasure, Draca's head came up, pointing in their direction. We knew he had no eyes or ears, and we thought he had no nose either, but he certainly had a nose for gold. He stayed head up, alert and motionless, for days. As soon as the warriors were gone he was off, slithering across the landscape, his body moving like waves on a duck pond, until he reached the mound. Draca just left us and took possession of the mound and its buried gold.

Draca jealously guarded the mound and its gold. It was his gold now, and he allowed nobody near it. If anybody went near the mound, and some brave souls tried at first, he would lash them with his tail, and they would scurry away with bruised behinds. Nobody could get near, not even Wynflaeth, no one but me; after all, he was my worm, or perhaps I was his. He still enjoyed me tickling his head, and he always did, right to the end.

We came to call the mound Draca's Dun, which means Dragon's Hill in our language.

It seemed like he somehow took energy from the gold which made him ravenously hungry. He took small creatures at first, mice and rats and hares living around the foot of the mound. He had a way of opening his mouth very wide and taking a creature whole, then sucking it down into his crop so he could digest it slowly. That was when his breath began to smell, with all that rotting flesh in his crop.

As he grew larger and larger he foraged further afield. That was when he started on our sheep. He would slither up to a grazing sheep, and before it knew what was happening Draca opened its great maw, and it was gone in a single gulp, sucked down into his crop. That was when we noticed he only took sheep, even ones with long horns, never rams; his taste was for females of any species he fancied.

The most terrible day was when he took Wynflaeth. She was sitting on her little three-legged stool under the cow's udder, grinning fondly at me and contentedly milking the cow into a big wooden pail. When Draca slid up she didn't take much notice; she was used to him being around. Only when he opened his great maw did she look alarmed. It happened so fast; one slurp and she disappeared.

I rushed at him, beating him with a stick, but it was hopeless; she was already in his crop. One moment she was there, so beautiful and fair a maiden; the next she was gone. Then Draca slurped the milk from the pail, slid under the cow's udder, and sucked her dry. I was so full of sadness and tears over losing my lovely Wynflaeth, and so cross with Draca, I wouldn't tickle his head for weeks.

After that, he had a taste for milk and maidens and would take no other. No maiden was safe from him; he could muscle his way across fields faster than any maid could run. Cows had no chance. Some maidens gave up being maidens to avoid becoming Draca's dinner, but it turned out he was not that choosy.

Draca grew really, really big on his diet of milk and maidens. If you go there now you can still see the deeply scored landscape where his great bulk slimed across it. When he wasn't foraging for his dinner he lay coiled around Draca's Dun, his vast tube of a body seemingly drawing energy from his precious gold, and with all those rotting maidens and sour milk in his crop, the stench of his breath was so disgusting, and what with his bad behaviour as well, he was known far and wide as the Laidly Worm.

The men decided something had to be done: a maiden a day keeps Draca away. They drew lots every day to see which maiden was to be Draca's dinner, along with six pails of milk. This put control back in our hands, they said. Typical! It was actually my father's idea; did I mention he was the local chief in charge of the hill fort?

So, every day a maiden was chosen by lot, her hands and feet were tied, and she was left with six pails of milk close to Draca's Dun, not too close on account of his abominable breath. One day it was my turn; it had to come even if I was the chief's daughter. Only the day before I'd been on the mound tickling his head. I'd had to forgive him for gobbling up Wynflaeth; it was just his nature after all. Now, there I was trussed up with six pails of milk and left there for his dinner.

As soon as he sensed who'd been left for his dinner he began to howl. He'd never howled before; I didn't know he could howl. He howled like he was suffering terrible anguish; well, I could see he was, howling and casting his great head from side to side. I could see he had a whole lot on his mind, him being my worm and all.

He was still howling when King Gaarge turned up, cantering slowly out of the misty west. As my mother said, she always gave herself airs, being a chief's woman.

He cantered up to me and got down from his horse.

"Call me King Gaarge," he said, "Scourge of dragon-kind. The dread news of your Laidly Worm has passed from mouth to mouth over hill and vale to my abode far in the west. Now I am here there is no more cause to fear." He'd get on well with my mother, I thought.

He looked about as much of a scourge as a stick of celery, but he did have this big sword which he liked to brandish as he strode about, going on and on about all the dragons he had slain, while I lay there trussed, with Draca howling and his noxious breath making the milk curdle.

Finally, he marched off up the mound, waving his sword. He had some pluck, I'll say that for him, clambering over the clammy coils. He'd never have got away with it if Draca had been himself; he'd have swallowed him whole and belched him back out, probably sword and all. But, poor Draca, he was in such torment over being given his own as his dinner he didn't see what was coming. With five swift strokes King Gaarge plunged his sword into each of Draca's five hearts, and it was all over for Draca. No contest. That's the true story.

Afterwards, King Gaarge boasted about his great victory over the Laidly Worm to anybody who wanted to listen, which was everybody except me. Only I knew about Draca's inglorious end, and nobody was interested in my story.

King Gaarge told them how he had leapt in to save the maiden, the chief's daughter even, as the dragon was about to devour her, how he had withstood the dragon's fiery breath, and how his experience as the scourge of dragon-kind had prevailed and he had struck the blow which brought the dread beast its demise.

So, that was the story which has been told ever since, of how King Gaarge slew the Dragon on Dragon Hill, and I can tell you, it's pure myth. I hope, after listening to my story, you'll credit what really happened; after all, I was there, the worm was mine, and I was his.

Sources

Newbury and District Field Club (1912); Simpson and Roud (2000), *A Dictionary of English Folklore*, see entry on 'dragons', pp. 110–111; Vinycomb, John (1906), p. 86.

Reflections

My Psychological Reflection

Another dragon tale? Another allegory? A narrative in which characters, places, and events can be interpreted to represent a meaning, in this case, with psychological significance.

The characters in this allegory are: milkmaid *Ethelinda*, meaning *Noble Snake*; sister *Wynflaeth,* meaning *Beautiful & Fair*; *Father*, the local Chief; *Mother*, who gives herself airs; *King Gaarge*, scourge of dragon-kind, who will go to any lengths to fulfil his vocation. And, of course, *Dark Demon Dragon Draca.*

Your Psychological Reflection

King Gaarge and the Dragon is a fun tale. It would be such a pity just to turn to the dark side of the story. So, instead, to keep up the fun, I shall set for you an allegorical puzzle. We can call the puzzle 'Everyone has a Serpent Inside.'

The characters in this allegory are: *Noble Snake*; *Beautiful & Fair*; *Father* the Chief; *Mother* with Airs; *King Gaarge* with a Vocation. Suppose these are parts of an *Ethelinda* personality, with *Draca* as the serpent inside. What do you know about these characters? What sense have you of their Bodily looks? Feelings? Thoughts? Spiritedness? What does your intuition tell you about *Noble Snake's* childhood? The story certainly unfolds, so how does it unfold for each of the characters? Whatever happens to *Beautiful & Fair*? From finding a worm coiled on her pillow, how does the reliance between *Noble Snake* and *Dragon Draca* develop? What does *Draca* represent? I have given you a couple of clues. Keep in mind, we are looking at aspects of the *Ethelinda* personality. Finally, here comes the plucky *King Gaarge*, and it's all over for *Draca*. How come? Have fun with the 'Everyone has a Serpent Inside' puzzle.

Mr Fox

A tale to be told to older children

'Mr Fox' is an English version of the French folk tale 'Barbe Bleue', 'Bluebeard', the story of a wealthy man habitually murdering his wives. I first heard the English folktale 'Mr Fox' as part of a workshop by the captivating Jennifer Westwood at the Society for Storytelling Annual Gathering in 2000.

I tell the story using my djembe drum, striking the drum twice every time I say 'Mr Fox'. I invite the listeners to join me; each time I say 'Mr Fox', I beat the drum and they shout 'boom-boom'. It's a bit chaotic but a lot of fun.

I told 'Mr Fox' at The Sir Donald Bailey Academy Primary School on Bailey Road, Newark, the home of the Bailey Bridge. I thought it a good idea to include the school percussion in the story, rather than the children shouting 'boom-boom'. I totally lost control, with 60 children all bashing away all the time, as I tried to shout the story above the hubbub. I apologised to the unamused staff.

Standing in the lunch queue later with a sympathetic headteacher, the two girls in front of us in the queue turn round and say to me, "Liked the stories, Sir." I ask, "Which story did you like best?" They reply, without hesitation and in unison, "Mr Fox."

A story can state an existential dilemma briefly and pointedly,
in a way which resonates with the listener's own inner conflicts,
so they can imagine themselves healed and being whole.

Synopsis

Lady Mary, being young and fair, has many suitors, the bravest and most gallant, and the richest, being the enigmatic Mr Fox. Before their wedding, while Mr Fox is away, Lady Mary seeks his castle home in the deepest, darkest part of the forest, there to discover, to her deliverance, his deepest, darkest secret.

The Story

Lady Mary was young, and Lady Mary was fair. Lady Mary had many suitors, but of all her suitors the bravest and most gallant, and the richest, was Mr Fox *{boom-boom}*. Lady Mary had met Mr Fox *{boom-boom}* when she had visited her brothers' house in the country. Nobody knew anything about Mr Fox *{boom-boom}*, or where he lived, or how he had gained his great wealth, but of all her suitors Lady Mary loved Mr Fox *{boom-boom}* best of all.

It came about that Lady Mary and Mr Fox *{boom-boom}* should wed. Sometime before the wedding, Lady Mary said to Mr Fox *{boom-boom},*

"Mr Fox *{boom-boom}*, where shall we live once we are wed?"

"Ah," said Mr Fox *{boom-boom},* "we shall live at my castle in the deepest darkest part of the forest."

A few days before the wedding, Mr Fox *{boom-boom}* said to Lady Mary,

"I shall be away for a few days on business."

So, Lady Mary decided that she would seek out Mr Fox's *{boom-boom}* Castle in the deepest, darkest part of the forest. When she finally found Mr Fox's *{boom-boom}* castle, the drawbridge was down, the gate was open, and over the gate she saw the words, 'Be bold, be bold.' Boldly, she walked through the gate into the courtyard, and over the doorway into the castle she saw the words, 'Be bold, be bold, but not too bold.' Not too boldly, Lady Mary went through the doorway into the castle. There she saw a grand staircase leading up to a long gallery. She climbed the stairs and walked to the end of the gallery. There she found a small door, and over the door she saw the words, 'Be bold, be bold, but not too bold, lest that thy heart's blood doth run cold.'

Lady Mary opened the door. Her heart's blood ran cold when she saw the bodies and bones of all Mr Fox's *{boom-boom}* previous wives covered in blood. Slamming the door, Lady Mary fled from the sight along the gallery and began down the stairs. Through the castle window, she saw Mr Fox *{boom-boom}* dragging a woman after him, and she was young and fair.

Lady Mary hid herself behind some wine barrels and watched as Mr Fox *{boom-boom}* dragged the poor woman, young and fair, into the castle, all the time trying to pluck a large diamond ring from her ring finger. With exasperation, Mr Fox *{boom-boom}* drew his sword, and with an upward strike he hacked off the young woman's hand.

Lady Mary stifled a gasp as the severed hand landed in her lap.

On the morrow, it was the time of the wedding. Mr Fox *{boom-boom}* was there. Lady Mary and her brothers were there. Lady Mary spoke to Mr Fox *{boom-boom},*

"Last night, Mr Fox *{boom-boom},* I had a dream."

"Well, my dear," replied Mr Fox *{boom-boom},* "why don't you entertain us by recounting your dream, as we await the time of our nuptials."

"In my dream," began Lady Mary, "I sought your castle in the deepest darkest part of the forest. The drawbridge was down, the gate was open, and over the gate I saw the words, 'Be bold, be bold.'"

"But, 'tis not so, and 'twas not so," chuckled Mr Fox *{boom-boom}.*

"In my dream," continued Lady Mary, "I went through the gate into the courtyard, and over the door to the castle I saw the words, 'Be bold, be bold, but not too bold.'"

"But, 'tis not so, and 'twas not so," declared Mr Fox *{boom-boom}.*

"In my dream," continued Lady Mary, "I went through the doorway into the castle, where I saw a grand staircase leading to a long gallery."

"But, 'tis not so, and 'twas not so," spluttered Mr Fox *{boom-boom}*.

"In my dream," continued Lady Mary, "I climbed the staircase and walk to the end of the gallery, where I found a small door, and over the door I saw the words, 'Be bold, be bold, but not too bold, lest that thy heart's blood doth run cold.'"

"But, 'tis not so, and 'twas not so," fumed Mr Fox *{boom-boom}*.

"In my dream," continued Lady Mary, "I opened the door and my heart's blood ran cold when I saw, Mr Fox *{boom-boom}*, the bodies and bones of all your previous wives, covered in blood."

"But, 'tis not so, and 'twas not so, and god forbid it should be so," raged Mr Fox *{boom-boom}*.

"In my dream," continued Lady Mary, "I fled along the gallery and down the stairs, and through the castle window I saw you, Mr Fox *{boom-boom}*, dragging behind you a woman, young and fair. I hid behind some wine barrels, watching as you dragged the poor young woman into the castle, all the while trying to pluck the large diamond ring from her ring finger, until in exasperation you drew your sword and hacked off her hand."

"But, 'tis not so, and 'twas not so, and god forbid it should be so," stormed Mr Fox *{boom-boom}*.

Lady Mary calmly replied,

"But, 'tis so and 'twas so," reaching into a fold of her wedding gown, "and here's the hand and ring to show," pointing the hand at Mr Fox *{boom-boom}*.

Lady Mary's brothers drew their swords and hacked Mr Fox *{boom-boom}* into a thousand pieces.

Sources

This story comes from *False Foxes*, compiled by Jennifer Westwood for the Society for Storytelling Annual Gathering, 2000, selection and notes © Common Knowledge 2000. Her attribution reads:

Mr Fox. From Joseph Jacobs, *English Fairy Tales* (London, 1890). The story was contributed to Edmond Malone's *Variorum Shakespeare* (1790) as an illustration of Benedick's remark in *Much Ado About Nothing* (Act I, Sc. i): 'Like the old tale, my lord, "It is not so, nor t'was not so, but indeed, God forbid it should be so."' Thus, *Mr Fox* was already current around 1600, when Shakespeare wrote *Much Ado About Nothing*.

Reflections

Egalitarian Reflection

'A tale to be told to older children?' Really? Writing this, I am appalled to think how often I have told children such a horrific tale of a serial wife killer. And how much they enjoyed it! Well, at least this serial wife killer gets his comeuppance. I even saw *Mr Fox* featured in a website for teachers, openly described as 'a tale of horror', even complete with an accompanying Teaching Pack. As a society we seem to be inured to violence.

Though *Mr Fox* has a history going back over 400 years, the story is really a contemporary horror story; according to the Femicide Census (www.femicidecensus.org/) at least 147 women were killed by 144 men in 2021. A total of 666 femicides—the number of the beast—occurred in the five years 2016–2020.

After this, dear reader, I hope you can endure re-reading the story as I have told it to children.

My Psychological Reflection

Like Bluebeard, Mr Fox is a serial wife killer motivated by financial gain and most likely hatred of women.

A *Psychology Today* article on serial killers (www.psychologytoday.com/us/blog/wicked-deeds/201909/understanding-what-drives-serial-killers) by criminologist Dr Scott Bonn, cites seven non-exclusive categories of motivation for serial killers: hostility toward a certain subgroup of the population, such as the homeless; criminal enterprise; financial gain; hatred of a specific gender or ethnic group; the feeling of empowerment or exhilaration; psychosis; and sexually based motivation. Serial killers "[a]re actually insecure individuals who are compelled to kill due to a morbid fear of rejection. In many cases, the fear of rejection seems to result from having been abandoned by their mother in early childhood. … Some serial killers are tormented, abused and even tortured by their birth mothers."

You are unlikely to have had a serial killer as a client, unless you've worked at "The Moor" (Broad or Dart). However, you may have a client referred to you to address uncontrolled bouts of violence, or more likely the wife of such a man. A man prone to bouts of domestic violence, though his behaviour is uncontrolled and dangerous, falls far short of being a serial wife killer. All the same, Dr Scott Bonn's article provides an indication of the origins of the man's psychological condition: an insecure individual unconsciously driven by a morbid fear of rejection, having been emotionally abandoned, and possibly also tormented and abused, by his mother in early childhood. This is evidenced by the mortification and remorse typically poured out to his spouse following a bout of violence. It is as if the man projects his desire for a longed-for-loving mother onto his wife, then something triggers him to project onto her his hated, rejecting mother.

Your Psychological Reflection

Here is an insecure man, unconsciously driven by a morbid fear of rejection, prone to bouts of domestic violence followed by an outpouring of mortification and remorse, who has found his way into your therapy room. How are you going to undertake therapy work with him? How would you portray his Soul? It seems evident that he has a violent part and a remorseful part, so would you consider doing parts work with him? How might you go about it? Once you had clarified the parts—how each part behaves, looks, feels, thinks, wants, needs, and the qualities lying beneath the behaviour—how might you approach the synthesis of these parts?

He is an insecure man, supposedly at the pre-personal stage of consciousness and will. How might you gently support and guide him to attain a personal self, with the self-awareness to become conscious of the childhood origins of his violent conduct, and the will to change his behaviour?

The Dun Cow of Parlick

Suitable for older children

With my brother Alan, I visit Bleasdale Circle, the Gathering Circle, below Parlick Fell in the Trough of Bowland. Bleasdale Circle is the site of an early Bronze Age wood-henge (See Figure below).[2]

I stand in the henge's outer circle. I enter a dream state, visualising myself standing with the villagers while the elders perform a ceremony within the inner circle, seeking wisdom from the Earth Goddess. I see one of the elders approaching me. He holds a spear horizontally towards me, between his outstretched fists, and looks into my eyes. Though I have never heard of this before, I know it is a sign of peace, friendship and welcome. I grasp the spear between my fists.

As everything begins in the imagination,
healing begins in the imagination.

Synopsis

At a time of famine in the area of Parlick Fell, an enormous dun cow appears with an abundant supply of milk. Each day she drinks by a well called Nick's Water Pot and allows anyone to take just one pot of her milk. One day, an old hag, a maker of ceramic pots, substitutes a sieve hidden in her cloak for her pot. The old woman milks all day, the milk flowing in a rich and copious stream. In vain the bountiful beast taxes her powers to fill the old hag's sieve. The fountain that had never failed at last runs dry. Whether of exhaustion or vexation or disappointment at being outwitted by the old woman, the dun cow returns from whence it came, but the people are saved.

The Story

A dark cloud gathered over the land. Crops wilted. Grassland withered. Sheep and pigs died. The people starved. The village folk flocked to the Gathering Circle for the ceremony of seeking wisdom from the ancestors and aid from the Earth Goddess. The Gathering Circle was on level, sheltered ground within a curve of fells, one of them Parlick Fell. The villagers gathered within the Circle's outer ring of 30 tall timber posts. The ceremony was performed by elders inside the sacred inner ring, where the cremated bones of the most ancient and wise ancestors were buried.

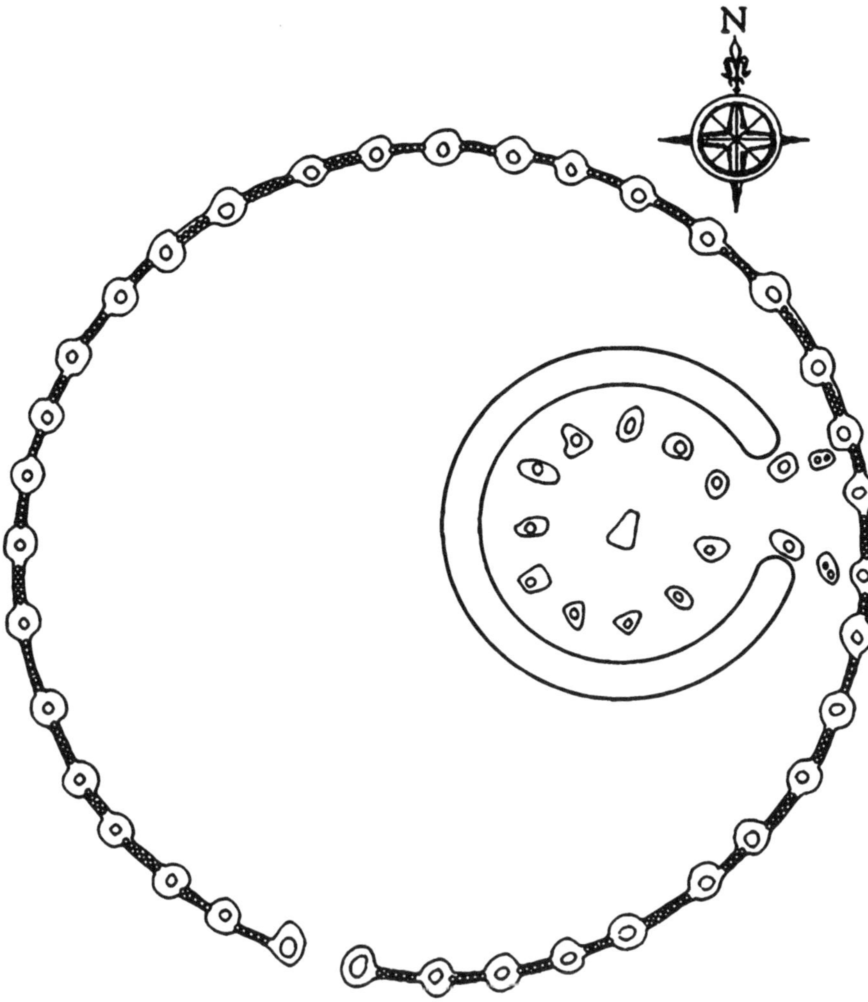

Figure 6.2 Bleasdale Circle Illustrator Terry Rushworth.

Opening the circle, the head man of the village held out his spear between his outstretched fists towards each elder in turn, to welcome and include them in the circle, each elder grasping the spear in acceptance.

The elders called on Serpent Spirit of the West, Wolf Spirit of the East, Bear Spirit of the North, Hawk Spirit of the South, and the Wisdom of the Ancestors to be with them in appealing to the Earth Goddess to aid the people in their plight.

As if in answer to their plea, there was a rumble in the nearby Parlick Fell, growing to a grinding roar of great stones grating together. The earth was in travail.

Parlick Fell heaved forth its progeny, a mighty beast, before the eyes of the people. It was a gargantuan cow, dun as the native stone and of the same stuff.

The ground shook beneath the Dun Cow's hooves as she trod the moor towards the Gathering Circle. She came to a stop just outside its outer ring, by a pool called Nick's Water Pot, from which she drank. With a sustained bellow reverberating across the landscape, the Dun Cow began to fill her colossal udder.

Then, she tossed her great head and swung her bountiful udder, a clear signal to the famished folk. They quickly brought their earthenware pots and one by one filled them to the collared brim with the Dun Cow's copious, creamy milk.

The Earth Goddess had answered the people's plea from her own body. The community was saved. Throughout the dark time, the Dun Cow came daily to Nick's Water Pot to drink, and the people brought their earthenware pots for a share of the Dun Cow's abundant bounty. But she only allowed each person one brimming pot. It was unbearable to the Dun Cow for anyone to try and fill another earthenware pot; she would shake her head and swish her tail with disapproval, and with a couple of quick kicks she would smash both of their earthenware pots, sending milk flying and the milker bruised and broken, then gallop off, tossing her head and kicking her feet in an agony of anguish and loathing.

Some time before, a strange woman had arrived in the village, tall and strong and dour, pulling a sled bearing a large pile of clay that she had prised from virgin earth. She told the villagers she had something marvellous to show them. She spent a day gathering straw, dry grass, and ash from the village fires. Then, she grabbed a hunk of thick clay and kneaded the clay into the shape she wanted it to be, a hollow log open at one end, then another, until she had a collection of 12. She placed the 12 clay logs in the sun.

The next day, she built a pottery kiln. She laid layers of straw and dry grass with the clay logs between and covered the heap with ash, leaving small holes at the apex and base. She took a brand and lit the straw from the base, then sat tending the heap for a day and a night. When the hole in the top had ceased to smoke, she slept by the heap for two days. When she awoke, she carefully took the heap apart, lifted out 12 earthenware pots, and showed them to the curious villagers. They looked at the earthenware pots in wonder, turned them over in their hands, and felt them with their fingers. They were amazed by the woman's magic, how she had changed hunks of clay into vessels that they saw instinctively how to use.

The mysterious woman remained in the village, though she always stayed aloof from the villagers. Soon, everyone was using her earthenware pots, although they viewed her magical power with awe and her with foreboding. Now, her earthenware pots were being used by the whole village to collect milk from the Dun Cow.

When the potter first approached the Dun Cow, she turned her broad head and glowered at the woman, her wide eyes dark with mistrust. The potter had made a vessel twice the depth and width of the villagers' pots. All the same, the Dun Cow allowed the potter to milk her, but the woman pulled on her teats roughly and with savage satisfaction. It was the same every day; the glowering cow allowed the potter to fill her oversized earthenware pot brim full, and the woman treated her with harsh and brutal disdain.

On the last day, the potter came to Nick's Water Pot in the late afternoon, when she could be alone with the Dun Cow. She placed her earthenware pot beneath the udder and began to milk. She had made this vessel with holes in the bottom. The bounteous stream of milk flowed through into a pot which could never be filled, Nick's Water Pot.

As her milk flowed and flowed, the cow gazed helplessly at the potter, with growing unease and distress as she became aware of the woman's enmity and malevolent design. The potter mercilessly milked on and on into the night, viciously drawing down the teats, with a widening sneer of malicious pleasure. When the udder became slack, she triumphantly stripped out the final drops. The Dun Cow's abundance was spent. She feebly kicked her heels and wandered over the darkened moor towards Parlick Fell.

The following day, when the Dun Cow failed to appear, the village folk flocked to the Gathering Circle to confer together and to consult the Earth Goddess. The elders opened the circle, calling on Serpent Spirit of the West, Wolf Spirit of the East, Bear Spirit of the North, Hawk Spirit of the South, and the Spirits of the Ancestors to join them in appealing to the Earth Goddess.

As if in answer to their plea, torrential rain began to fall, lightning filled the dark sky, and there was a thunderous rumble on nearby Parlick Fell, as of great stones tearing apart. The Earth Goddess was taking back her own. The rain ceased. The dark cloud cleared. The sun shone. The villagers in the Gathering Circle saw that spring was nigh. For these people, it was as if the Dun Cow had never been.

Sources

Grice, Frederick (1953); Harland, John & Wilkinson, T. T. (1873); Harris Museum and Art Gallery, Bleasdale Circle Leaflet. Harland & Wilkinson tell us of an old farm at Whittingham, five miles north of Preston, named the 'Old Rib' because, mounted over the door, was the enormous rib of the fabled dun cow.

First published in Lancashire Folk Tales (Jennie Bailey and David England, 2014).

The pottery kiln I describe in the story is based on the traditional kiln I saw in use at Durbar Square—Pottery Square—in the medieval city of Bhaktapur, Nepal (see potterysquare.com).

Reflections

My Psychological Reflection

I preceded *The Dun Cow of Parlick* tale with an account of my visit to Bleasdale Circle in the Trough of Bowland, the site of an early Bronze Age wood-henge. In writing this reflection, I find that I need to include my experience at the Bleasdale Circle as well as the tale itself.

When I visit some ancient sacred site, I can have a waking dream, like my presence at the village ceremony to seek wisdom from the Earth Goddess, often including surprising images, like the elder holding out a spear between his outstretched fists as a sign of welcome. For me, a waking dream is simply a way of bypassing the constraints of my conscious mind so as to access my unconscious mind, what I prefer to call my inner world of imagination and wisdom.

Subsequent to my visit to Bleasdale Circle, I trained in a technique for accessing the inner world of imagination and wisdom as a psychotherapeutic method, the practice of the shamanic journey, with its origins in the ancient Siberian 'technique of ecstasy'. *Woo-woo!* Don't get too excited. In traditional shamanism, the technique of ecstasy is the ability to leave the body and travel in the spirit world (Eliade 1964, p. xix), or, in present-day parlance, travel to the inner world of imagination and wisdom.

A shamanic journey is like a dream, with two significant differences. Firstly, a person enters the journey with an *intention* to explore a specific topic, maybe some seemingly intractable problem. Secondly, they can remember the journey afterwards and report what occurred. Grounding the traveller's experience of the journey and reflecting on its significance for their life is an essential part of the psychotherapeutic process of the shamanic journey. I drum throughout a journey. A drumbeat of 4Hz or 240 beats/minute, corresponding to theta waves in the brain, helps the traveller to relax and to remain in a dream state.

A full account of the shamanic journey can be found in my book *Soulfulness: The Marriage of Shamanic and Contemporary Psychology* (England 2017, pp. 83ff). A CD *Drumming for the Shamanic Journey* is available at *Eagle's Wing Centre for Contemporary Shamanism* (https://eagleswing.co.uk/), where I did my Shamanic Journey and Medicine Wheel training.

Much of the time as a writer, my creative process is to gain insight from my inner wisdom, an overall sense of what I am trying to write, before my conscious mind can compose the right words. I make a shamanic journey with the *intention* of gaining insight into what I am trying to write, to the sound of a 20-minute drum CD.

Now, I find I spontaneously descend into a dream state at other times when I am relaxed. At night, sometimes in a dream, sometimes half waking from sleep, especially when awakening in the morning, and sometimes out of the blue, I receive an intuition pertinent to my current writing. Clients have sometimes reported a similar phenomenon.

In the middle of last night, I entered a dream state. Here's what came to mind. Someone said recently, "The transpersonal is no better than the personal." It's true. Receiving insight from my inner world of imagination and wisdom is a gift of grace. Yet, for a gift of grace, I can take no credit personally. It's transpersonal.

My Transpersonal Reflection

As I dream my way into *The Dun Cow of Parlick*, I begin to realise how I had failed to recognise, much less understand, the fraught relationship between the old potter and the Dun Cow, the woman's enmity and the cow's mistrust. The story now has a deeper meaning for me, about the tension between the natural world and the products of human ingenuity. The gargantuan Dun Cow, a product of the earth, is a positively nourishing boon to humanity until her finite resource is spent by the old potter, who drains and strips her. At the same time, the people are reliant on the old potter's earthenware pots in which to collect milk from the Dun Cow.

The story serves as a metaphor for the world today. Like the villagers of Bleasdale, we are caught in a dilemma. We are heavily reliant upon the products of human ingenuity, many of them brilliant inventions, whilst these products serve to strip the planet of its finite resources. In 1972 I visited the offices of Bolt Beranek & Newman (BBN) in Cambridge, Massachusetts, to learn about ARPANET—The Advanced Research Projects Agency Network—which BBN had been contracted to develop for the US Department of Defense. ARPANET became the technological foundation of the Internet. That the Internet is a massive boon to billions needs no explanation, yet it places weighty demands on the world's energy resources with significant impact on global warming, with further colossal demands since the introduction of AI.

I could have included this story in the Transpersonal Tales Room.

Your Psychological Reflection

If you are a writer or involved in another creative activity, I wonder, what is your creative process? How do you make a connection with your unconscious, your inner world of imagination and wisdom?

To what extent do you access your inner wisdom in your therapy work? In a therapy session, there is an outer space and an inner space. The outer space is your connection with your client, seeing them, listening to them, and paying attention to them. The inner space is your connection with yourself, your conscious mind recording what unfolds and maintaining an overview of the session, and your inner wisdom giving you intuitive insights into what is unfolding and the interventions you might make.

I invite you to reflect on your experience, in your therapy work, of your outer space and inner space, and your access to intuitive insights from your inner wisdom.

The Great Hairy Toe

Suitable for older children

This is one of the few American tales in my collection and is one I love to tell because there is so much listener participation, even a choice of ending.

Synopsis

A scruffy old woman who lives in a deep, dark wood is on her bony knees, foraging for mushrooms and whatever else she can unearth, when she finds a great hairy toe. Reassured that the great hairy toe is not attached to a great hairy beast, she returns to her hovel and, with enormous relish, fills her belly with great hairy toe soup, then contentedly retires to her narrow bed. In the middle of the night there comes the distant sound of tramping in the wood and a distant voice calling, "I want my great hairy toe." The sounds come nearer and nearer until … Well it doesn't look like there's going to be a happy ending for Old Bony Knees, but you never know. Actually, there are two endings, so you decide which one you like, probably what most choose. Shame on you!

The Story

Once upon a dark time, a bony old woman lived in a dirty hovel in the middle of a deep, dark wood. She was not a nice person. Her frock was stiff with muck and grease. Her face was covered in blackheads. Her hair had never been washed since, well, ever really; even nits wouldn't nest in it. Her long, thin nose had a flattened end with large, bristly nostrils, more a long, thin snout than a nose.

The old woman lived on roots, which she dug up in the wood, mushrooms, and sometimes truffles when she could find them. Every now and then she found flesh to eat, maybe a dead stoat or a rabbit stolen from a trapper's snare.

One day, she went into the wood as usual to collect food in her old wicker basket. She knew the best spots, bending down and snuffling in the undergrowth with her long snout, sniffing out the softest roots and plumpest truffles. Suddenly, in her snuffling, she smelt an unfamiliar odour. Rummaging in the leaf mould with her long, bony fingers, she found a hairy toe, a great hairy toe.

Down on her knees beside the great hairy toe, the old woman said to herself,

"Where there's a great hairy toe there's likely to be a great hairy foot. And where there's a great hairy foot there's likely to be a great hairy person. Or even a great hairy beast." She began to be afraid. Cautiously, not daring to look up, she felt around the great hairy toe but could find no great hairy foot, nor any great hairy leg, nor any great hairy beast attached to it. Feeling a little bolder, she squeezed the great hairy toe between her finger and thumb and sniffed at it. It felt nice and plump and smelt fairly fresh.

"Mmm!" she said to herself, and smacking her flabby lips she popped the great hairy toe in her basket with the roots and mushrooms and the odd truffle.

When she returned to her hovel, she took the great hairy toe out of her basket and tipped the roots and mushrooms and the odd truffle into a cauldron with onions and herbs and lots of oil and garlic and water from the butt. Then she placed the great hairy toe, almost tenderly, into the pot and placed it over the fire. Soon her bristly nostrils smelt with delight the delicate odours of great hairy toe soup.

The old woman ladled the hot hairy toe soup between her flabbily smacking and slurping lips, over her yellow tongue and chomping gums and down her gurgling gullet. She plunged her bony fingers into the cauldron to grasp chunks of tender toe. Lifting them high and throwing back her nit-less head, she threw the morsels in the air, caught them in her toothless gums, and after a few munches swallowed them with a loud,

"Glumph!" She spent a few rapturous moments with her fingers in her mouth, sucking and plucking out hairs from the great hairy toe caught between her gums.

Then, grasping the cauldron between her greasy hands, she opened her gullet and poured the rest of the great hairy soup straight down into her stomach. Wiping her greasy fingers on her greasier frock she let out a sustained and contented belch and climbed the stairs to her narrow bed.

The old woman pulled the blanket up to her neck and fell into a satisfied sleep. In the middle of the night there came a distant sound out there in the deep, dark wood. It went tramp-ramp, tramp-ramp, tramp-ramp. As the tramping and ramping became louder the sound pierced the old woman's slumbers. She awoke with a shudder, pulling the blanket up to her ears. Tramp-ramp, tramp-ramp, tramp-ramp. Then a voice to accompany the tramping and ramping,

"I want my great hairy toe. Where's my great hairy toe?"

The tramping and ramping got nearer and nearer, tramp-ramp, tramp-ramp, tramp-ramp, and the voice got louder and louder,

"I want my great hairy toe. Where's my great hairy toe?" until they had almost reached her porch. The old woman leapt from her bed, ran down the stairs, bolted the door with a heavy iron bolt, and then ran back to her bed, pulling the blanket right over her head.

The heavy door burst from its hinges with a crash which shook the hovel to its sparse foundations, the iron bolt broken asunder. There was a stretched moment of utter silence. Then, a great voice was in the house,

"I want my great hairy toe. Where's my great hairy toe?" and a tramping and ramping was on the groaning stairs: tramp-ramp, tramp-ramp, tramp-ramp.

By now the old woman was under the narrow bed, her heart pounding like a tight drum in her hollow chest, her unblinking eyes fixed on the bottom of the bedroom door, which ever so slowly began to creak open. Then, she saw, crossing the threshold into the room, two great hairy feet and one great hairy toe, with a light tramp-ramp. She heard, in a menacing whisper,

"I want my great hairy toe. Where's my great hairy toe?"

Peeping out from under the bed, the old woman saw, attached to the great hairy feet, great hairy legs, and attached to the great hairy legs, just a great hairy mouth, a mouth on legs. The great hairy mouth had leering looks and a lolling tongue, a savage sneer and snapping jaws. Its breath foul as a hen hut, it breathed,

"Where's my great hairy toe?"

At this moment, the great hairy toe, the one inside her stomach that is, began to rumble, revealing the old woman's hiding place. The great hairy toe, the one still attached to the great hairy foot, poked the old woman out from under the bed. The great hairy mouth breathed again,

"Where's my great hairy toe?"

"Um!" cried the old woman, "You can't have it. I um! I et it."

> *{Now, there are two ends to this story. You, the reader or listeners, can decide which one you prefer.}*

The first ending:

"You et it?" hissed the great hairy mouth, "Then, I shall just have to eat it back." The great hairy mouth leant down towards the old woman with widening jaws, then nothing could be heard but the crunch of brittle bones. Then, nothing could be heard. And nothing was heard of the old woman ever again.

The second ending:

"You et it?" hissed the great hairy mouth, as it leaned down towards the old woman, where she lay. And gave her a great, sloppy kiss.

She looked up at him with a satisfied look, saying,

"What shall we play tomorrow, Henry?"

> *{It's surprising how often children prefer the first ending. Or maybe not.}*

Source

This story is based on a traditional tale from American folklore, *The Hairy Toe*. I have not been able to find its source, though it seems to have been collected by S.E. Schlosser, author of a series of 'Spooky' tales from around America.

Reflections

Egalitarian Reflection

Honestly, it's just a story; I'm not getting at bony old women. In truth, I always go for the second ending, so romantic, such a charming couple, and her saucy question, "What shall we play tomorrow, Henry?" shows how it is she who calls the shots in their erotic games.

My Psychological Reflection

I thought I'd just included *The Great Hairy Toe* in this Room because I like it, because I love to tell it in all its gross detail, and because it's a lot of fun. I now realise, humour is one of the humane psychological attributes of the right hemisphere (Iain McGilchrist, 2009). Come to think about it, in my therapy room there's a little weeping and a lot of laughter, even in the midst of sorrow.

Your Psychological Reflection

How much laughter is there in your therapy room? Oh, never mind, just enjoy the story and have a laugh.

Lady Sybil and the Milk White Doe

Suitable for older children

> *This story is one of the oldest in my repertory, from long before I included it in Lancashire Folk Tales, and I have a deep love for it.*

The story is the healer; the story touches the Soul.

Synopsis

Lady Sybil lives, and loves to roam, on the high, wide moor, learning its secret lore, but has no eyes for the besotted Lord William, who fears she will be accused of witchcraft. He consults a wise old crone, her left leg trailing slightly as they walk together around her herb garden. After hours of bandying words with him, she finally guides him on what to do. When the moon is full and high, he looses his hounds on the moor. They pursue a milk white doe, who easily outpaces all the hounds, save one, a craggy old bitch with a game hind leg, which Lord William fails to recognise, and who holds the doe's hind leg gently in her jaws till he catches up. He throws a silken cord about the doe's neck, leads her to his home of Hapton Tower, and locks her in a stately tower room. In the night, the tower is battered by stormy winds. When Lord William unlocks the tower room door, there he finds Lady Sybil, combing her hair. Soon they are wed, though this is not the end of Lady Sybil's excursions on the moor, when the moon is full and high, accompanied by her constant companion.

The Story

Lady Sybil lived in an ancient tower on the high, wide moor, hard by the promontory of Eagle's Crag. Lady Sybil possessed charm and grace, beauty and wit. She had many suitors, not least of whom was Lord William of Hapton.

Although Lord William showed her unfailing love and devotion, Lady Sybil had no eyes for him. Her love was for the wild moor. Her greatest pleasure was to pace the hills by day, and, on such a night as this, when the moon was full and high, to stand upon Eagle's Crag, gazing upon her.

During her lonely moorland walks, Lady Sybil felt more and more drawn to becoming a woman wise in the lore of the land. She studied herbs and potions and tried them upon herself. On such a night as this, when the moon was full and high, she lay in the bracken by Eagle's Crag and gazed upon her until her senses reeled and she became entranced. In her trance, she became a rabbit and a stoat. She became hare and harrier. She became lark and hawk, pigeon, partridge and plover. She became gorse and heather, couch grass and fern, tormentil and wild thyme. But her greatest joy, on such a night as this, was to become a milk white doe, a pale streak racing across the high, wide moor, or standing upon Eagle's Crag, framed against the moon and calling to her. Thus she learnt the secret lore and language of the earth.

Lord William kept watch on her from a distance, with grief and longing in his heart and growing anxiety in his guts, fearing she was losing her wits, and worse, through her practice of witchcraft she might lose her life at the end of a hangman's rope. As he kept watch, not daring to interfere, there grew in his anxious mind the idea of rescuing her from herself.

Lord William consulted an aged crone who lived in those parts. She was a healer and a wise woman, but she was also feared as a witch by superstitious folk.

"Set a witch to catch a witch," was Lord William's maxim.

He met the crone in her herb garden, harvesting fumitory and thyme. Her face was as ancient, craggy, and full of character as the harsh high moorland landscape in mid-winter. Her huge knuckles stood out from her gnarled hands. Her left leg trailed slightly as she walked around her herb garden.

When Lord William had told the crone of his fears for Lady Sybil, she invited him into her cottage, which was neat, warm and comfortable. A potion was bubbling on the open range, filling the cottage with delicate aromas of sage and sandalwood. Around the shelves were the crone's herbs of healing, many with animal names: cat's ears and mouse ear; cowslip and oxlip; chickweed, cuckoo pint, and bird's foot trefoil; hogweed and sowthistle; toadflax and wormwood; harebell, henbit, and hawkbit; foxgloves and bats in the belfry.

Lord William haggled with the crone for hours, urging her to persuade Lady Sybil to desist from her dangerous pursuit of wisdom. The lord's cogent arguments the crone deftly deflected, for they disregarded the passion in the lady's heart. The threats to the lady's life the crone treated with disdain, for they discounted the lady's will and calling. The lord's desperate offers of wealth the crone rejected with contempt, for they were a slur upon her own integrity and calling.

The crone let the lord exhaust himself of all his arguments, threats, and bribes. Then she told him what he must do,

"On such a night as this, when the moon is full and high, take to the moor with your best hounds. You will start a milk white doe from cover. Pursue her, but do not kill or harm her. When you have caught her, bind her loosely about her neck with a silken cord and lead her gently to your manor. Then sleep, and leave the rest to me."

On such a night as this, when the moon was full and high, Lord William took his hounds to the moor and loosed them. The hounds snuffled in the bracken and gorse until they started from cover a milk white doe, which sped away from them, a pale streak racing across the high, wide moor, leaving the hounds far behind. All save one, which the lord failed to recognise, a craggy old bitch with a game hind leg, which kept with the milk white doe pace for pace.

With bursting lungs and aching legs, Lord William caught up with the milk white doe as she stood by Eagle's Crag, framed against the moon and calling to her. The craggy old bitch held the doe's hind leg gently between her jaws. He threw a silken cord about the doe's neck and led her to his home of Hapton Tower. He felt she was too fair a creature to leave in a stable, so he locked her in a stately tower room hung with fine tapestries. Then he went to his couch.

Barely had Lord William sunk into an exhausted sleep after his exertions on the moor, when he was abruptly cast from couch and slumber as a great storm blew up, battering against his home, and Hapton Tower began to rock on its foundations. Worthy ancestors fell from walls, fine porcelain toppled and smashed on the tiles, pots and pans crashed onto the kitchen floors, dressers burst open scattering family silver, and chained hounds howled with fear and anguish in their kennels.

Struggling out of a tangle of sheets, Lord William made for the tower room where he had left the milk white doe. Often he was flung against the walls, as the building rocked and tilted, or thrown down to grovel among the shards and silver, tearing his legs and hands. Bruised and bleeding he reached the tower room. As he unlocked the door, the shaking and quaking of his home subsided as suddenly as it had begun. The door swung slowly open. Instead of the milk white doe, there was Lady Sybil, naked and at ease, quietly combing her pale tresses.

Soon after, Lady Sybil and Lord Hapton were wed. They had many children. Each day Lady Sybil walked the high, wide moor collecting herbs, often with animal names. Her family never ailed, but she had a potion or poultice to soothe and heal them. And on such a night as this, when the moon was full and high, her soul would soar out onto the high, wide moor, where she would lie in the bracken by Eagle's Crag and gaze upon the moon. Entranced, she became the creatures of the moor. Best of all, she became the milk white doe, standing at Eagle's Crag, framed against the moon and calling to her.

So, whenever the moon is full and high, if you have the eyes for it, you can see her still, a pale streak racing across the high, wide moor, or standing upon Eagle's Crag, framed against the moon and calling to her. And at her heels, you can see her constant companion, a craggy old bitch with a game hind leg.

Sources

Grice, Frederick (1953); Harland, John, & Wilkinson, T. T. (1873).
First published in Lancashire Folk Tales (Jennie Bailey and David England, 2014).
The Lady Sybil Legend is also recorded in the Hapton Heritage website, www.haptonheritage.co.uk/the-lady-sybil-legend/.

Reflections

Egalitarian Reflection

There is only one thing to say. Lady Sybil is the finest exemplar of mature, wise, self-willed womanhood.

Your Psychological Reflection

I invite you to read *Lady Sybil and the Milk White Doe* again, carefully and reflectively, phrase by phrase. Then, read the 'Reflections' on *The Dun Cow of Parlick* story. Then, lie down with closed eyes and dream your way into *Lady Sybil and the Milk White Doe*, with the intention of discovering Lady Sybil: as having a mature ego with the will to survive in the world; as having attained a personal self, with a capacity for self reflection and the will to make life choices; as having a transpersonal self with increasing realisation of being willing to be part of the whole, along with other people and other living things; as touching your Soul.

My Psychological and Transpersonal Reflection

I could have included *Lady Sybil and the Milk White Doe* in the *Transpersonal Tales Room*. Lady Sybil is at the transpersonal phase of her psychological journey. Heedless of her own safety, she sees beyond herself to the secret lore and language of the land and her fellow creatures, creatures of whom she is one and with whom she is at one.

The Witches of Windsor

In this beastly tale, it is people who are beastly. The accused old women, healers and midwives, show compassion towards their principal detractor, and in their final hours they conspire to save his soul. I could have included this story in the Transpersonal Tales Room.

I set out to tell this tale from the perspective of the accused women, but when I read about the discovery of wax images in the women's homes, with the accusation of treason and witchcraft, I felt stumped and my writing slumped. Then, during lunch on a shamanic training weekend at Compton Dundon in Somerset, I overheard someone at the other end of the table speak of corn dollys—that's it, corn dollys, not wax images—and the tale untangled itself.

A contemporary account by John Alde (1579), 'A brief treatyse conteyninge the most strange and horrible crueltye of Elizabeth Sule [sic] alias Rockingham [sic] and hir confederates executed at Abington upon Richard Galis,' is considered to be a testimony by Richard Galis, who had accused the women of witchcraft.

The story is the healer
and serves as a container for each listener's Soul energy.

Synopsis

In Elizabethan Windsor, four impoverished old wise-women, Elizabeth Style, Mother Margaret, Mother Deuell and Mother Dutton, are accused of witchcraft by Richard Galis. The discovery of three wax images, with thorns through their hearts, in a London dung heap, brings their case to national prominence when similar images are found in the homes of the accused witches. The three images are thought to represent Queen Elizabeth and two privy councillors and are therefore treasonable.

In the furore which follows, the four women are arrested and imprisoned at Reading. Elizabeth Style makes a detailed confession that she and the three others accused used their 'familiars', a toad, cat, and rat, to bring about the deaths of prominent Windsor citizens and some cattle. After being tried and convicted, they are hanged at Abingdon on 28 February 1579.

The Story

My name is Elizabeth Style, and this is my tale. Though, I confess, not the tale I told the gaoler at Reading before the trial. The tale's not only about me and my sister wise women. It's also about three poor demented souls, Master Richard Galis and his sons Richard and James.

I'm sitting in a dank prison cell in Abingdon, with my friend Margaret and two other old women whom I've always known as Mother Deuell and Mother Dutton. We've been condemned to be hanged as notorious witches. Strangely, as wise women we have no truck with witchcraft—it is our superstitious, frightened detractors who believe we employ such power.

My dear old friend Audrey Seidre would have been here with us, if Master Richard Galis hadn't had this frail old woman manhandled into church in front of the congregation. She died, God rest her soul.

Audrey and I grew up together. We watched and learned from our mothers as they worked. They were healers and midwives. They were wise in the lore of the land, the frailties of human bodies, and the mysteries of childbirth. We were destined to follow in their footsteps.

The wisdom which our mothers gave us has been known to our female forebears for numberless generations, a wisdom rooted in the time of the old religion, when every plant was seen to possess an enlivening spirit. For, how else would plants know to reach out to the sun, or trees know when to bud.

Our forebears unearthed the secret quality of every plant to heal body and soul. We've inherited this wisdom. Alas, in more recent times, the uprooting and supplanting of the old religion has put women like us in peril. When folk need our help in sickness, they turn to us. When they're taught to see us as part of the old religion, they demonise us and accuse us of witchcraft.

Our herbs often have animal-like names: toad flax for problems passing water, cat's ears for jaundice, and yellow rattle for women's problems. We give our patients the names of the herbs we use. It's reassuring when we show how familiar we are with their use. If only we'd known how our words would be made to turn and bite us! Our accusers claimed we had 'familiars', devils in the form of toads, cats, and rats, to help us carry out our evil deeds.

As midwives, we're admitted into the mysteries of women's bodies, matters men are ignorant of, arousing in them fear and envy, suspicion and distrust. Besides, childbirth has many hazards which threaten death to mothers and babies. Aye, we can share a mother's joy at the nativity of a healthy child, but when it goes wrong we can suffer rancour, rage, and blame.

Our work's mostly been for the poor folk of Windsor. We're paid what little they can afford for healing their diseases and bringing their children into this world. After all that, we end up living in hovels and alms-houses and finally being hounded to our deaths.

Our troubles began some years ago. Mother Dutton was summoned by a distraught Master Richard Galis, thrice Mayor of Windsor, saying his sons, Richard and James, were possessed by devils. Mother Dutton has a rare gift of seeing deeply into the soul. In Richard and James she saw immense suffering and heartache as well as brimming rage. She treated them both, as she told Master Galis, with a strong dose of chase-devil.[3]

James failed to respond to the treatment. Instead, his rage boiled over, pouring out obscene curses on Mother Dutton, throwing stones at her house, shouting accusations of witchcraft, and calling her "mother" and "witch". Then, he became totally still, his body frozen into a rigid pose, his hand twisted back upon itself. He went completely mad, crying unceasingly,

"Away with the witch," and had to be confined.

Young Richard claimed he'd been visited by the apparition of a huge and mighty black cat, creeping towards him from the shadows of midnight, filling him with fear and dread. Nevertheless, he seemed to respond well to treatment, better able to cope with his afflictions. Yet, he too focused his rage on Mother Dutton and became hell-bent on her destruction, indeed, the destruction of us all.

Master Galis sought vengeance on Mother Dutton for James' madness. He said she had promised to use chase-devil to chase the devils out but instead had invited more in. He dragged her before the mayor, Richard Redforth, on a charge of witchcraft. Knowing Master Galis' temperament, Master Redforth ordered Mother Dutton released forthwith.

Galis stormed off, lamenting 'the lack of better magistrates to weed out such malefactors'. Undaunted, shortly afterwards he seized Mother Dutton, as she made her way to Clewer, where she lived in a straw house, and dragged her to Windsor gaol. The gaoler, with a knowing shake of his head, refused to take her in without a warrant from the mayor.

Unrelenting, Master Galis then abducted Mother Dutton, Mother Deuell, Audrey and me, and delivered us to the country house of his friend Robert Handley, who had lost the use of his legs and believed himself bewitched.

Galis demanded we cure Handley's bewitchment on the threat of being cudgelled. Matters then became confused. Handley insisted we recite the Lord's Prayer and quizzed us on the Ten Commandments. The outcome was that a half-crazed Galis was taken into custody, manacled, and imprisoned, so the gaoler told us, in a deep dungeon he was lowered into on a rope. He was held without bail, charged with abduction and false imprisonment.

Alone in his dark cell, deprived of human company or even a bed, he began to fear he would die there, but after two days the mayor relented and released him. Of course, he alleged we used our familiars to incense the mayor against him and effect his imprisonment. When he later died, his raging son Richard accused us of bringing about his death, calling us 'these hellhounds and imps of the devil'.

Richard then became our main detractor, though he often had bouts of lunacy, seeing black cats and fiends with fiery eyes. Once, he tried to burn down Mother Dutton's straw house by thrusting a cloth dipped in brimstone into it and lighting it with a brand, but the straw was too wet.

The next few years were quiet, on the whole. There were mutterings against us when two butchers, Switcher and Mastlin, died of the plague on their return from London. There was trouble when an ostler refused to pay me after his wife had a stillbirth and again after Mother Deuell had spirited away a neighbour's monstrous birth. Richard Galis made various attempts to raise funds after his father died, but his temperament made him unfit for trade, and they turned sour. Then, he bought some cattle and sheep, but they were poor stock that mostly died. Of course, in his poor, tormented mind, he saw us despoiling his purse and stock by witchcraft.

During this time, we met Father Rosamond of Farnham Royal. His real name was Osborne, but he decided to change it and to set himself up as a cunning man after his wife died. She was a wise woman of great skill, and her daughter has followed in her footsteps, a highly intelligent and perceptive young woman. She's well versed in herbal lore, which she wisely kept hidden from her father. We've tried to keep her name out of all this, so she can continue her good work in peace.

Rosamond asked us to meet him at the marling pit behind Master Dodge's property, but all he wanted was to learn a few tricks from us. We refused, and I reckon he bore a grudge.

Living beneath the walls of Windsor Castle, news filtered down to the townsfolk that Queen Elizabeth's agitation about Catholic plots against her is much intensified since her excommunication by Pope Pius V. Like most people in these times, she's deeply superstitious. She's terrified of being killed by witchcraft. So, matters became much worse for us when three wax images with thorns piercing their hearts were found in a London dung heap, representing, it was thought, the queen and two privy councillors. This was seen as treason.

Richard Galis now had his chance. He searched our homes and claiming to have found wax images hidden there, accused us of treason and witchcraft. Wax images, indeed! They were just corn maidens. Women in our families always helped with harvest and made corn maidens from the last sheaf of corn to hold the spirit of the corn goddess until she was ploughed back into the earth to ensure a good harvest the next year.

Galis seized me, tied a rope around me, and dragged me through the streets of Windsor to the Castle, to the jeers of the townsfolk. He arrested Margaret and Mother Deuell, but when he went for Mother Dutton she locked herself in a chest and mocked him from inside. However much he fumed, he couldn't get her out, while the fickle crowd ridiculed him. It would've been funny if it hadn't been tragic.

After this affront, Galis had a fit and stormed off to Father Rosemond's home.

"I'm tormented," he said, "by infinite pains in body, and by purse ache." He dragged Rosamond out by his hair, wielding a cudgel, and furiously demanded the man cure his ailment. Rosamond cried out,

"You are bewitched," and identified me, Mother Dutton, and Mother Deuell, as the cause.

Well, the Privy Council appointed the Dean of Windsor, Sir Henry Neville, to find out if we had plotted to kill the queen by witchcraft. Faced with this impossible task, all he could do was examine us on our religious education, which was precious little, and make us sit beneath the pulpit, in front of all the people, during the service. Then, he sent us to Reading for trial. I was still a strong woman and walked all the way without discomfort, but after the treatment I received at Reading gaol I could barely stand.

As we four old wise women sat together in Reading gaol, we knew there was no hope of justice for us. Everybody, from the queen downwards, was in an implacable grip of fear and a frenzy of superstition. They needed scapegoats. So, here we were, weak, frail old women, fearing further torture to force confession.

Yet, we felt a quickening strength and power in us, the only power left to us, the power to heal. We chose to confess the most heinous and villainous enchantments and witchcraft. Yes, partly it was to end the torture, but mainly we had a deeper intent. By holding up to Richard this mirror of his false mental attitude, he might thereby come face to face with himself, face the truth of his own calumny, and find healing for his soul.

I opted to be the one to make a 'confession' to the gaoler, on behalf of us all, in the presence of Richard Galis, while the other three giggled and sniggered like mad old women: conspiring to murder Master Galis and the butchers Switcher and Mastlin by enchantment and the use of familiars; conspiring to cause James and Richard Galis to be possessed by devils; conspiring to despoil by witchcraft Richard Galis' herds and to cause him purse ache.

The trial was quickly over, and we were brought to Abingdon by cart with a deeply pensive Galis riding alongside. As we trundled along, we sang:

Alas, my love, ye do me wrong
to cast me off discourteously:
And I have lovèd you so long,
Delighting in your company.
I have been ready at your hand,
to grant whatever you would crave.
I have both wagered life and land,
your love and good will for to have.[4]

As we sang, our words slowly penetrated Richard's mind and pierced his heart. His rage left him. His eyes cleared. For the first time, he saw the whole picture, the injustice which his mad rage had inflicted. Upon his face we saw understanding dawn, chagrin rise, and remorse and sorrow surface. But, however much he now desired it, he could not prevent the relentless wheels of Justice trundling towards the gallows.

Now, our work is done. We shall have a song of thanksgiving on our lips and in our hearts all the way to the scaffold, the threshold of our life beyond.

Sources

Alde, John (1579); Kupfermann, Elias (2011); Matthews, Tony (2011); White, Edward (1579)

First published in Berkshire Folk Tales (David England and Tina Bilbé, 2013)

Note

Gallys Road in Windsor is named after Richard Gallys, a prominent Windsor resident and Mayor in the 16th century who was the landlord of the Garter Inn and is believed to be the inspiration for the character of the host in Shakespeare's *The Merry Wives of Windsor*. Gallys Road is located in the Dedworth area of Windsor.

Reflections

Your Psychological Reflection

What was Elizabeth Style's purpose in 'confessing' to the crimes of which she and the other two women had been accused?
Who do you think is the central character in this story, and why?
What might it have been like for Richard Galis to have his accusations mirrored back to him?

My Psychological Reflection

The Witches of Windsor is a story of selfless love. "There is no greater love than this, that someone should lay down his life[5] for his friends." (Revised English Bible, John 15:13). There is no greater love than this, that after a life of service to others, three old women lay down their lives for their tormentor.

Notes

1 Illustrator Jo Lowes.
2 Illustrator Terry Rushworth.
3 St John's Wort.
4 From Greensleeves.
5 Or her life.

Bibliography

Alde, John (1579) *Pamphlet 'A Brief Treatyse Conteyninge the Most Strange and Horrible crueltye of Elizabeth Sule [sic] Alias Bockingham [sic] and hir Confederates, Executed at Abington, upon Richard Galis,' Bodleian Library Reference: 'Gough Berks. 1'*.
Bailey, Jennie and England, David (2014) *Lancashire Folk Tales*, The History Press.
Eliade, Mircea (1964) *Shamanism, Archaic Techniques of Ecstasy*. Arkana Penguin Books.
England, David (2017) *Soulfulness: The Marriage of Shamanic and Contemporary Psychology*. Routledge.
England, David and Bilbé, Tina (2013) *Berkshire Folk Tales*, The History Press.
Grice, Frederick (1953) *Folk Tales of Lancashire*, Thomas Nelson.
Harland, John, and Wilkinson, Thomas Turner (1873) *Lancashire Legends, Traditions, Pageants, Sports, etc.*, George Routledge. Manchester: L. C. Gent.
Kupfermann, Elias (2011) *Article 'A Case of Witchcraft in Elizabethan Windsor' in Windlesora 27*, Windsor Local History Group.
McGilchrist, Iain (2009) *The Master and His Emissary: The Divided Brain and the Making of the Western World* (p. 190), Yale University Press.

Newbury and District Field Club (1912) *Excursion to Tom Hughes' Country—Uffington, Kingston Lisle*, White Horse Hill, Waylen Smith's Cave, Donnington Priory.

Schlosser, S. E. *A Series of 'Spooky' Tales from Around America.*

Simos, Miriam (Starhawk) and Valentine, Hilary (2000) *The Twelve Wild Swans: A Journey Into Magic, Healing, and Action*, Harper Collins.

Simpson, Jacqueline and Roud, Steve (2000) *A Dictionary of English Folklore*, see entry on 'dragons', pp. 110–111.

The Witches of Windsor, A Community Play, performed as part of the Windsor Arts Scene in November 2011, unpublished.

Vinycomb, John (1906) *Fictitious and Symbolic Creatures in Art*, Chapman and Hall.

Westwood, Jennifer (2000) False Foxes, Compiled for the Society for Storytelling Annual Gathering, 2000, Selection and Notes © Common Knowledge.

White, Edward (1579) *Pamphlet 'A rehearsal both straung and true of hainous and horrible actes committed by Elizabeth Style, Alias Rockingham, Mother Dutten, Mother Devell, Mother Margaret, Fower notorious witches, apprehended at Winsore in the Countie of Barks, and at Abington arraigned, condemned and executed On the 28th daye of February laste, Anno. 1579*', British Library Reference: c.27.a.11.

Beastly Tales Annex: 'Witches'

Egalitarian and Scientific Reflection

Wise-Women

In olden times, when you were ill or injured, you would have gone to a wise woman for treatment. She would have knowledge of the healing qualities of plants, minerals, and water, knowledge passed down from mother to daughter. She may also have used spells and charms to calm a troubled breast.

Christian Witch Theory

In the 16th century the Christian church became a threat to wise women, who were dubbed as 'witches' and as the Bible clearly states, "Thou shalt not suffer a witch to live (Authorised Version, Exodus 22:18)." Thus, there emerged the Christian Witch Theory: a wise woman must have gained her healing power by making a pact with the devil. Wise women were arrested, tortured to obtain confession, then mutilated, hanged, burnt at the stake.

Scientific Approach

Hot on the heels of the Christian Witch Theory, there came a further threat to the work of wise women, the advent of a scientific approach to healing, boosted by the founding in 1660 of The Royal Society to support scientific medical research. Though wise women, with their long experience of healing the sick and injured, might have made a significant contribution to medical discovery, they were excluded, only men being allowed to train as doctors.

For more information visit:

www.museumofcambridge.org.uk/wise-women-traditional-cures-and-remedies/.

DOI: 10.4324/9781003712329-9

Harvard Medical Student Review

The benefits wise women might have brought to the scientific development of medicine is revealed in a paper published in the Harvard Medical Student Review: 'What's in the Cauldron: Witches, Folk Remedies, and Their Contributions to Modern Medicine.' The full text of the paper is available at, www.hmsreview.org/issue6/2022/3/whats-in-the-cauldron-witches-folk-remedies-and-their-contributions-to-modern-medicine.

This academic paper examines retrospectively the effectiveness of wise-woman remedies, with an illuminating conclusion. There follow the Abstract, Conclusion, and Acknowledgement.

Abstract: Disease is a part of the human condition and before the rigour of the scientific process and peer review, healers had to work with anecdotal folk remedies and word of mouth medicines. These folk remedies were often known by women and shaman who, throughout time, passed on their esoteric knowledge. Some of these remedies, like excretions from toads, Hemlock, Yew, and Foxglove have persisted for centuries and were used for a wide range of ailments. In modern days, with the use of the scientific process and peer review, these plants form the foundation of many medications. This demonstrates the benefit that can be gained with the investigation of folk medicine.

Conclusion: Many medical advancements can be made by examining what is "in the cauldron". Witches and shaman, with their concoctions and folk remedies, have treated illnesses and ailments for thousands of years. The historical concoctions created in their cauldrons have greatly influenced the modern medical field. From the disgusting excretions of amphibians, roots of the Hemlock, bark of the Yew, and beautiful petals of Foxglove, we have taken what once seen as sorcery and turned it into medicine. Some of these remedies went thousands of years without an understanding of how they worked, only that they worked. Without the "witches" who used them, we may have never known or discovered their usefulness.

Acknowledgement: From: Harvard Medical Student Review. Author: Mason Tate Bennett, BS, Trinity School of Medicine, St Vincent and the Grenadines. Title of Article: What's in the Cauldron: Witches, Folk Remedies, and Their Contributions to Modern Medicine. Issue No: March 24, 2022. Copyright © 2022 Harvard Medical Student Review. Reprinted with permission.

Bibliography

Bennett, Mason Tate (2022) What's in the Cauldron: Witches, Folk Remedies, and their Contributions to Modern Medicine' *Harvard Medical Student Review*, Issue No: March 24, 2022.

Transpersonal Tales Room

The transpersonal goes beyond a person's capacity for self-reflection to a sense of intimate self-reflexive consciousness, of other human beings, of other creatures, of the world of nature, and of the world we live in.

The Work That Reconnects

Joanna Macy, veteran environmental thinker, writer, teacher, and campaigner, designed a groupwork programme 'The Work That Reconnects' to foster the desire and ability of people to take part in the healing of our world. The programme is informed by Deep Ecology, systems thinking, Gaia theory, and spiritual traditions. 'Joanna Macy and Her Work' is further described on the website www.joannamacy.net/main.

Central to the programme is the recognition that the basis of choice-making is self-reflexive consciousness; self-reflexive consciousness can realise The Great Turning, the shift from the Industrial Growth Society to a life-sustaining civilisation. This is transpersonal.

'The Work That Reconnects' is continued by Molly Young Brown, co-author with Joanna Macy of 'Coming Back to Life'. Molly Young Brown brings Psychosynthesis and Ecopsychology into the programme. 'Molly Young Brown' and her work are further described on the website https://mollyyoungbrown.com/

The story is the healer.

DOI: 10.4324/9781003712329-10

Tales for the Great Turning

I was invited to provide an evening of storytelling for the local 'Great Turning' group, who follow the work of Joanna Macy. I named the storytelling performance 'Tales for the Great Turning' and gathered this collection of stories with an environmental context: our connection with the natural world; rainbow, sun, and sky; and the elements of water, earth, air, and fire.

It feels important for me to stress that these are stories with an environmental context; they are not stories with a moral. The listener or reader needs to be free to take what they need from a story, not to be preached at. I abhor stories with a moral.

Psychological Reflection on These Transpersonal Tales

During my psychotherapy training, I received a verbal Year End Report, "You'll be alright up till two." What could that mean?

I reckon, the prospect of acknowledging to ourselves that we have reached the transpersonal phase stirs up those childhood admonishments about not being boastful, at least with me. As therapists, we need to be able to recognise where our centre of gravity is; with our clients, we'll be alright till then. We need to be able to acknowledge when, on the *Journey of Becoming*, we are in the transpersonal phase and have humility about it, else we are just in a game of snakes and ladders.

The transpersonal phase of human life is in the recognition that one is not separate from the time/space continuum, which is the whole of existence. While once existing as stardust, one is not separate from the sun and stars from which one came, not separate from the elements—water, earth, air, fire—existing within and without one, not separate from one's seed flowing back in time to the first self-reproducing organism, not separate now from other people, other species, nor from responsibility. Such self-reflexive consciousness is what we as therapists need to seek if we are to help our clients to find it. The issues addressed in these transpersonal tales are the issues our transpersonal clients are concerned about.

Dream Dilemma

> *I recently experienced the joy of connection with another species in a garden planted with buddleia to attract butterflies, watching close-up as peacocks, red admirals, marbled whites, and cabbage whites supped nectar from the flowers.*

As everything begins in the imagination,
healing begins in the imagination.

The Story

Zhuangzi dreams he is a butterfly, struggling to get free from the chrysalis. He squeezes from the chrysalis and opens his wings for the first time, a beautiful pattern of red and orange and blue, flecked with white and yellow. He is enthralled.

A draft of wind arises under his wings and he soars into the sky, learning to shift his wings to match the breeze. He has always wanted to fly. Now, he alights on a leaf, closes his wings and opens them, closes them and opens them again, such wonder.

A bright yellow sunflower catches his eye. He feels an urge to fly down onto the sunflower, to sink his proboscis into the flower, to sup the sweet nectar like a straw, to savour such richness of flavour, aah!

Then he awakes. He touches his lips. He ponders, "Am I a man who dreams he is a beautiful, enchanted butterfly. Or am I a butterfly, dreaming I am a man? Is there a difference?"

Source

Zhuangzi is the name of a great Chinese philosopher who lived around the 4th century BCE in the Meng province, present-day Henan. You can find the story at:

www.thechinastory.org/yearbooks/yearbook-2019-china-dreams/forum-illusions-and-transformations-the-many-meanings-of-meng-%E5%A4%A2/zhuangzi-and-his-butterfly-dream-the-etymology-of-meng-%E5%A4%A2/

Our Psychological Reflection

This Room starts and finishes with stories about human connection with another species. *Dream Dilemma* expresses the joy of feeling a sense of union with the natural world. For the therapist, it is enthralling to be present as a client squeezes from the chrysalis and opens their wings for the first time.

The Three Golden Hairs

Suitable to tell or read to older children

> *'The Three Golden Hairs' is a glorious anthropomorphic myth about the rising of the sun.*

We sin against the imagination when we ask a story for its meaning.

The Story

A moonless night, pale starlight filtering through the canopy, a frail, white-haired old man making his painful progress through the forest, his legs faltering, his thin arms drawing him slowly forward from tree to tree, the creaking of his bones answering the screeching of night owls, his lantern burning low, making his way towards a distant light.

At the end of his strength, he comes to a low cottage, through its window the welcoming, flickering firelight illuminating his path. Reaching the door, he is spent, snuffing out like his lantern, collapsing on the threshold.

Rising from her chair by her cosy fire, an old woman, wise and strong, gathering up the old man, carrying him like a bag of bones to her chair by the warm fire, and gently holding him through the night, rocking him like a baby,

"There, there! There, there!"

The dark of night on the edge of ebbing into twilight, the old man transforming into a fine-looking young man of strengthening limbs and golden hair, the wise old woman still gently holding him, rocking him,

"There, there! There, there!"

Approaching dawn, the wise old woman gently holding in her lap a beautiful young child, his locks like ripening wheat, then plucking three golden hairs from the child's head, dropping them on the hearth tiles with a ting, ting, ting, releasing the child from her lap; he runs to the door, turning to give her a warm smile before leaping into the sky, the bright morning sun breaking over the forest.

Source

I have no record of where I found this myth, and I have failed to discover it online. If you know, please, tell me.

Our Psychological Reflection

Ting, ting, ting! This little tale awakens us to our neighbourhood star, our shining Sun, the source of all life's energy, which evolves and sustains us and all the richness surrounding our planet.

Glorious it may be, but I strain my brain to discern what this deceptively simple story might tell us. An old man, his energy spent at the end of the day, is gently comforted and his life energy revived by morning by a wise old woman, at the price of three precious hairs.

I don't like to interpret tales, yet I feel I'm getting uncomfortably close to interpretation when it speaks to me of the revitalising outcome from tending a life crisis. What does the tale suggest to you?

Tiddalik the Frog: In the Dreamtime

A tale to be told to young children

> *The story is set in the Dreamtime, the time before time, for Aboriginal people the spiritual beginning of all things: rivers, streams, waterholes, the land, hills, rocks, plants, and animals. And it's a story for children, who are a living embodiment of the natural cycle of life.*
>
> *'Tiddalik the Frog' is a lovely story to tell interactively with children ages 4-8, set out here in the way I tell it, with my interjections. I could have included it in the Storytelling With Children section.*

Let the story tell the story.
The story enables the listener to generate a new way of experiencing themselves, which at the outset is unknown.

The Story

Tiddalik lived in the time before time. He was a frog, a big frog, a very big frog, a very, very big frog.

{How big? very, very big.}

The soles of his feet were so big he crushed whole forests as he walked through them.

Tiddalik was thirsty, very thirsty, very, very thirsty.

{How thirsty? very, very thirsty.}

He opened his mouth and swallowed whole clouds of rain. He swallowed up all the rivers, drained all the lakes and pools, and even slurped up all the puddles. He grew an enormously fat belly with all that water inside him.

The other animals were gasping for water.

{I grasp my throat and gasp for water.}

The plants were wilting, and the trees were dying. The animals didn't know what to do until Wombat suggested,

"Let's have a meeting."

It was a gloomy meeting …

{I pull a silly gloomy face.}

… with everybody saying, between gasps,

"We're done for, we'll never get Tiddalik to give up his water."

Then Wombat came up with another idea,

"We'll make Tiddalik laugh so that he splurts all the water out."

{I make a squirting raspberry.}

The animals weren't gloomy now; they all wanted to try and make Tiddalik laugh. So they all went off to where Tiddalik was sitting with a long face, thinking about water.

{I pull a long face.}

The first to try was the laughing Kookaburra.

{I make a Kookaburra laugh (look it up on the internet). Try being a Kookaburra.}

The other animals rolled about laughing.

{Did Tiddalik laugh? NO-O! Did he titter? NO-O! Did he grin? NO-O! Did he smile? NO-O! Not even a twitch? NO-O!}

Tiddalik just sat with his long face.

{I pull a long face.}

The next one to try was Kangaroo, bouncing up and down, BOING, BOING, BOING.

{Did you know, it was Kangaroo who invented the trampoline?}

The other animals rolled about laughing.

{Did Tiddalik laugh? NO-O! Did he titter? NO-O! Did he grin? NO-O! Did he smile? NO-O! Not even a twitch? NO-O!}

Tiddalik just sat with his long face.

{I pull a long face.

I invite the listeners to try other animals to make Tiddalik laugh, and each time…}

The other animals rolled about laughing.

{Did Tiddalik laugh? NO-O! Did he titter? NO-O! Did he grin? NO-O! Did he smile? NO-O! Not even a twitch? NO-O!}

Then another animal slithered up. It was Eel, and he was in a worse state than the other animals because the pool he swam in had been swallowed up by Tiddalik. Eel wanted to have a go.

"Well," said the other animals, "you might as well, we haven't made him laugh." Eel gazed up at Tiddalik. Eel began to sway, rising up on the end of his tail.

Then he began to dance, da-da-da-dada-dada-dada-da, dadada-da-dada-dada-da.

{Did you know, it was Eel who invented the snake dance? I sway about and dance to the rhythm da-da-da-dada-dada-dada-da, dadada-da-dada-dada-da.}

The other animals gazed at Eel's antics in awe. Tiddalik's eyes turned to Eel. Tiddalik's mouth began to twitch. Then he smiled a little smile. Then Tiddalik grinned. Then Tiddalik tittered. Then Tiddalik laughed, rolling about clutching his enormous belly, and all the water splurted out of his mouth, filling up the puddles, and pools, and lakes, and rivers. All the animals could at last quench their thirst.

It was Wombat's idea. It happened in the dreamtime.

{Give yourselves a clap for being such wonderful storytellers. We all clap. }

Source

I found *Tiddalik the Frog* in a charming little book, *The Music and Story Experience with Pippa Reid*, a storytelling friend, with original illustrations by her daughter Rachel Reid. The book contains Pippa's version of this Australian Aboriginal tale.

Our Psychological Reflection

Tiddalik the Frog is a tale about the element of water. Water is essential to life, our own and that of other species. We are one with the element of water, for each of us is around 60% water. The scarcity of fresh water is a growing issue in our present world. We need to learn to conserve and share water, not fight over it, which means putting aside self-interest and working together, which means more and more of our species to move into the transpersonal phase, in which as therapists we may see ourselves as in the vanguard, not in a crusading way, but in the quality of our work.

The King and the Oak

> *'The King and the Oak' is about the element of earth, into which trees and plants plunge their roots, upon which we ourselves are rooted, and which for us is a metaphor for groundedness.*

The right story holds up a mirror to the listener's existential experience, and it is this which brings healing and transformation.

Synopsis

There was a beautiful sacred oak grove watched over by Demeter, goddess of harvest. In every tree there lived a tree-nymph, the lives of tree and tree-nymph interwoven. Near the sacred grove, there lived a mighty and prosperous king, who decided to build the greatest palace there had ever been. He needed the tallest trees to support the mighty roof. He took 20 woodcutters to the sacred grove, giving no thought to the sanctity of the place. In the guise of an old priestess, Demeter warned him against offending the goddess of harvest. In reply, he took an axe to the grove's greatest oak, ordering his woodcutters to cut down every tree. When the king's new palace was completed, the land became barren, hunger entered the king's fine palace, his servants fled, and only the king and his daughter remained. The king sold his daughter into slavery for a crust of bread and flagon of water. When these were gone the mighty king died an agonising death. The sacred grove remains forever barren.

The Story

Erysichthon King of Thessaly had some reason to think highly of himself, king of a region of wide plains, watered by a wide river, abundant with cattle and crops. He thought to himself, I shall built a palace befitting my power and might, grander than any other, its roof span wider than any in the world, made of the mightiest oak timbers. Where would he find such timbers? His lips curled with derision as his mind turned to a sacred grove of ancient oaks in a nearby valley, where the great goddess Demeter had her temple.

In Demeter's sacred grove, the oaks had grown for centuries undisturbed. In each oak tree a tree-nymph lived in peace, for Demeter allows no axe to enter the grove. The life of a tree and tree-nymph were entwined; when a tree came to the end of its span of years and died, the tree-nymph also died. Demeter's sacred grove was a tranquil place, where pilgrims came for soul refreshment and Demeter's gentle care.

Erysichthon cared nothing for that. He ordered 20 woodcutters to sharpen their axes and follow him to the sacred grove. Heedless of the sanctity of the place or the alarmed rustling of the trees, he commanded the woodcutters to set their axe to every tree. The woodcutters, so overwhelmed by the sanctity of the sacred grove and in such shock at what they were expected to do, were too petrified to raise their axes. Consumed by rage, Erysichthon, grabbing one of the axes, plunged through the grove to its centre where stood the mightiest oak. As he raised the axe, Demeter, in the guise of an old priestess, appeared at his side, warning of how unwise it was to affront the great goddess Demeter. With a sneer he brought down the axe, plunging it into the heart of the oak. The tree-nymph's scream of anguish and pain resounded throughout the grove as it was taken up by her sister tree-nymphs. The traumatised woodcutters' will was broken, and they complied with the king's angry threats, chopping down and hauling away every tree.

Erysichthon was proud of his magnificent new palace, where he lived with his daughter Mestra in opulent splendour, heedlessly derisive of Demeter's warning. Meanwhile, Demeter, goddess of harvest, bided her time, allowing the king to lull himself into a false sense of security. Gradually, the wide river found other banks to flow between, other wide plains to water. Crops began to fail. Cattle began to die. Peasants took their remaining livestock to other lands. Hunger entered the grandest palace in the world. Servants filtered away until only Erysichthon and his daughter Mestra remained. They relied on passing caravans for food and water in exchange for precious palace objects. When all was gone, Erysichthon sold his daughter into slavery for a hunk of bread and a flagon of water. The mighty king soon died of hunger and thirst in mortal pain. He suffered the consequences of affronting the great goddess Demeter.

The valley where the sacred grove once stood remains forever barren. Even Demeter cannot restore the sacred grove of oak.

Source

This story is based on a Greek myth, told by Callimachus, *Erysichthon and the Grove of Demeter*, to be found at www.greeklegendsandmyths.com/erysichthon.html. Another retelling can be found at Alida Gersie, 1992. From *Earthtales, Storytelling in Times of Change.*

Our Psychological Reflection

It is astonishing that deforestation is the subject of an ancient Greek myth, when today the deforestation of our primeval rain forests is a matter of such deep concern. Then and now, it is ruthless greed that poses the threat. Then again, maybe we need to ask ourselves the question, how much am I culpable, consuming the products of deforestation, food crops, feed crops, fibre crops, and the rest? I'm shocked and don't know the answer myself! Well, I do know the answer.

Iris—Rainbow Goddess

The story of Iris is about the element of air; how Iris' alchemical transmuting of air and water and sun realises a spectral rainbow bridge spanning the sky, a symbol for humankind of hope and promise.

The story is the healer
and serves as a container for each listener's Soul energy.

Entranced

It is a cold November day. Overcast and gray. Yet, as I wander into Shepherd Market, a small London square, I step into warm sunlight from a cloudless sky. The air is light and balmy, rich with the flavour of oriental spices. I enter the intense life of the square. People laughing, talking, drinking, eating, browsing, buying, selling, playing music, kissing, loving it all. There are busy stalls selling bric-a-brac, old books, wooden dolls, and overflowing falafels with hummus in pitta bread.

Best of all, there is a rainbow of heaped spices, vibrant in the sun: red chillies, orange cinnamon, yellow turmeric, green wasabi, blue poppy seed, and even a purple chilli from Turkey with an unpronounceable name.

A rainbow! I realise with a jolt of insight—Iris is here. Iris, the Rainbow Goddess, is of all the ancient and immortal gods the one with most affinity with mortal folk. I am entranced.

The Story

Iris, she alone of all the gods, rides the rainbow. While Helios, the sun god, rides his horse-drawn chariot across the sky, and Hermes, messenger of the gods, has his winged sandals, Iris sails her chariot, drawn by a pair of dazzling peacocks, casting her radiant rainbow where she will. The Rainbow Goddess plays wherever she lets the light of the sun or moon illuminate the misty clouds and waterfalls.

Iris, whose name means both rainbow and messenger, is the messenger of the gods, bringing nectar to the Olympian gods and succour to humankind.

Iris' mother is a cloud-nymph, and her father is a god of the sea; she bridges sea and sky. She replenishes rain clouds, amassing droplets of water from the sea. She gathers rays of sunlight, deftly reflecting, refracting and dispersing the light in water droplets, to realise the radiance of the rainbow. She roots her rainbow earth to earth, her grand ethereal arch spanning, embracing, the sky, one glorious arc, then two, then three, to the delight of humankind.

Afterglow

The images fade. I return to a rare sight, a rainbow of heaped spices, vibrant in the sun: red chilies, orange cinnamon, yellow turmeric, green wasabi, blue poppy seed, and purple chilies. With a light heart, I leave the street market and step out of the small London square.

It is a cold November day. Overcast and grey. Yet, my heart sings.

Our Psychological Reflection

Rainbow, lightly evanescent as a whiff of fragrance, ephemeral as feeling, an epiphany of pleasure.

The Tiger and the Strawberry

A tale to be told or read to older children and adults

This is a serious story about the elusive nature of human happiness.

When I received my Diploma in Psychosynthesis Psychotherapy, I used it as my speech. My son Ed used his version of the story as the Introduction section of his MA thesis in Built Environment Studies, 'Life and Death: Unsettlements' (2006).

It's also a rollicking good story to tell to children, as I hope my version shows.

A story can state an existential dilemma briefly and pointedly,
in a way which resonates with the listener's own inner conflicts,
so they can imagine themselves healed and being whole.

Synopsis

Shankaracharya's Ātmabodha (see *Source*) introduces this story, "To illustrate the elusive nature of human happiness, Buddha narrated the vivid story of a man who, while roaming in the forest, was discovered and hotly pursued by a tiger."

The Story

A man is strolling in the forest, contemplating the meaning of life, wondering what the meaning of life might be, when he sees, bounding down the track towards him, an enormous tiger, with an even more enormous grin on its face, licking its chops.

Putting aside his contemplations, he hot-foots it in the other direction. As the tiger closes upon him, the track comes to an end at the edge of a cliff, and without pausing for reflection, lest he become a little light lunch, he launches himself into the void, AHAAAA!

With good fortune, he is able to grab hold of a vine, which brings him up short, SMACK! against the cliff face. The tiger is quite put out, and putting out its claws reaches down to where the man hangs, grazing the top of his head.

Once he has regained his presence of mind, he decides to look down, where he sees some good news and some bad news. The good news is that the bottom of the cliff is only a few feet below him. The bad news is that there is another tiger with its paws up the cliff, about to take a lunge at him. He pulls his legs up as far as he can so that this tiger is only able to graze the soles of his feet.

While thinking to himself, thank goodness for the vine, two little mice, a black mouse and a white mouse, creep out of a hole and begin to gnaw at the root of the vine. He decides it is time to make a general appraisal of his situation, with a hungry tiger above grazing his head, a hungry tiger below grazing his feet, and two voracious mice making his hold on the cliff face increasingly shaky, and he says to himself, another fine mess you got me into.

At this point, he notices, a short distance from him along the cliff face, where a shaft of sunlight breaks through the forest canopy, there is a strawberry bush. And, on this strawberry bush there is the biggest, reddest, juiciest strawberry he has ever seen. In his extremity, he reaches out, plucks the strawberry, and puts it into his mouth. Ah!, he says to himself in delight, absolutely delicious!

And that, he says to himself, that is ... that is ... where this story ends.

Source

I found this story on page 2 of the Hindu work *Ātmabodha*, meaning Self-Knowledge, by Shankaracharya. This is my loose retelling of this traditional story told by the Buddha.

Our Psychological Reflection

At the end of the film *Monty Python's Life of Brian*, the lead character has been crucified. A character on an accompanying cross tries to cheer him up by singing *Always Look on the Bright Side of Life*. As the song progresses, 23 other crucifixion victims appear on the screen, each dancing on their crucifix as credits roll.

In the therapy room with a suffering client, I wouldn't try to cheer the client up. I'm not sure I'd sing *Always Look on the Bright Side of Life*, but I might do something similar. Most likely I would invite the client to sit with me, together in the suffering, for us to await whatever meaning in the suffering may emerge.

A Woman Made of Salt: A Traditional Spiritual Story

Having unearthed this story from my files, I wondered about its source, where had I found it? I looked it up on my browser, which led me to an out-of-date page of my own earlier storytelling website, and there is was, clearly marked—© David England, 2003—along with its original source.

The story is the healer.

The Story

A long time ago... Or, a long time hence... Or, a long time now... There was a woman made of salt.

The woman lived beside the Great Ocean, the eighth ocean of the world. As time went by, she felt herself drawn more and more to the Great Ocean. She longed to plumb its depths and to know its span.

One day, she stepped into the Ocean. It covered her ankles, her knees, her thighs, and her vulva. As she immersed herself deeper and deeper in the Ocean, being made of salt she began to dissolve. She immersed herself more deeply in the Ocean. It covered her buttocks, her belly, her back, her breasts. More and more she dissolved in the Ocean, salty as she was. She immersed herself more deeply in the Ocean. It covered her neck, her face, and the crown of her head. For a moment her salt hair floated upon the Ocean, until it too began to dissolve.

And as the last particle of her dissolved, she became one with the Great Ocean. She knew its depth and span. Afterwards, even if she could, she would not return.

Source

This tale is based on a Vedantist Salt Doll parable told by Sri Ramakrishna (1943), "In samadhi one attains the knowledge of Brahman."

Our Psychological Reflection

This tale depicts the ultimate realisation of self-reflexive consciousness.

My Lord Bag of Rice

A tale to be told to older children

This is the last story I selected for the Collection, in place of one I felt didn't really fit. I used to tell 'My Lord Bag of Rice' a lot but had forgotten what an unusual tale it is, and so full of graphic imagery beloved by storytellers. Moreover, only now have I come to appreciate the psychological truths hidden within the fabric of the story. The landscape of the story reflects my experience of Nepal's Annapurna Trail, a narrow trail with a sheer mountain on one side and on the other a precipice into a roaring torrent, interspersed with precarious suspension bridges. Where the trail widens out, there are hamlets with fertile terraced hillsides and welcoming guesthouses.

Synopsis

A warrior, servant of the sun god, gathers his scimitars, a great bow, and all his courage to set off on a quest to right wrongs. He faces a fearsome dragon, which turns out to be a grieving old man, the Dragon King in the guise of a dragon. The Dragon King is beset by a horrific beast, who has grown fat on the bodies and souls of his sons and daughters, his grandsons and granddaughters, a centipede.

"A centipede!" I hear you cry. And so the battle commences.

The Story

This story takes place thousands of years ago, long before Siddhartha Gautam seated himself beneath the bodhi tree and Buddhism came to the land. A time when the people of the land practised the ancient religion of earth and sky; and even today, in remote hamlets, the people still practise that same religion, setting a white stone in the earth at the centre of each paddy field, "In honour of the goddess," I was told, "and to ensure the fertility of the crop."

In that land there lived a warrior, a servant of the sun god. The warrior—like warriors of every age and land—liked nothing better than to go on great quests, righting wrongs. He would go out from his village armed with a great bow and with two keen-edged scimitars at his belt. The scimitars were so sharp, his favourite party trick was to take a woman's hair and split it longways with a scimitar's edge.

One day, the warrior buckled his twin scimitars to his belt, slung his great bow on his back and set off on his quest. After many adventures, he made his way up a deep, wide gorge. The people who lived in this valley had terraced the hillsides. Their tiny fields reached high up the steep hills, wherever there was a patch of earth which could be terraced and cultivated.

Below him, as he walked, the warrior could see a river meandering through the stony floor of the gorge. Its waters were a pale green, the colour of jade. He came to a place where a great bow in the river had hollowed out a deep and silent pool. Beyond the pool was a high, conical mountain, its sides terraced almost to its crown. Below the pool, a long bridge hung in a high catenary above the river, giving access to the other side. The wooden slats of the bridge were whitened in the sunlight. The high, bright noonday sun reflected in the pale jade of the pool.

It was a rich and tranquil scene. Except, the warrior noticed, the terracing of the conical mountain was broken and the little fields uncultivated. A wisp of smoke drifted up from the mountain's crown. And a scaly dragon blocked his way across the bridge.

The dragon's foot clawed the wooden parapet of the bridge. Its forked tail lashed the parapet on the other side. Between, the coils of its body curled across the slats of the bridge. Smoke and flame drifted lazily from the dragon's nostrils as it eyed the warrior menacingly.

Undeterred, the warrior drew his twin scimitars and closed upon the dragon. Not that they would have been of any avail against such an adversary with its fiery breath and armoured hide. Steadily, he scaled the rough scales of the dragon's body, knowing, at any moment, the dragon might turn its monstrous head and with a single fiery breath burn his life to a cinder. Then, he was over the dragon's horny back and stepping down the other side. Gingerly, and with long strides, he stepped over the coils of the dragon's body as it lay across the bridge, knowing, at any moment, the dragon might tighten its coils and squeeze the last breath from his body.

Then, he was past the dragon, walking over the slats of the bridge to the other side, with measured tread, not looking back. He heard a quavering voice behind him, "Warrior!" and more loudly, "Warrior!" Turning, the dragon was gone, and in its place an old man, his back bent and his face lined with grief. Upon his whitened head there was a dragon crown.

"I am the Dragon King of the river lake," said the old man. "Long have I lain across the bridge in the form of a dragon, waiting for a warrior with courage enough to overcome its fearsome nature as you did. I can take the fiery form of a dragon, but I do not possess its power. I need you, warrior, to right the wrong which is being done to me and my family. I need you to slay my enemy, who comes nightly to the river lake and carries off one of my sons, my daughters, my grandsons or my granddaughters."

"I am bound by my oath to the sun god," replied the warrior, "to take up the cause of one who is ill-used by another and to right wrongs. But who is your enemy?" "My enemy is a centipede," said the dragon king.

{"A centipede!" I hear you cry.}

"A centipede!" echoed the warrior. "But this is no ordinary centipede," explained the dragon king, "This is a centipede who has grown fat on the bodies and souls of my sons and my daughters, my grandsons and my granddaughters. Soon, none will remain and I too will perish."

The warrior agreed to undertake the quest, and the Dragon King led him into his domain beneath the waters of the river lake. As the waters closed around him, the warrior was astonished that his clothes remained dry and not only was he able to breathe, but the air had a sweeter and livelier quality than the cold, dry air of the gorge. They entered the Dragon King's palace of white marble, with its tall turrets and balconies rising to just below the surface of the river lake, commanding a clear and secret view of the conical mountain.

The Dragon King honoured his guest with a fine feast served by goldfish and red carp and silvery trout; crispy lake weed, freshwater anemones in sweet and sour, lemon rice and crystallised lotus flowers in stem ginger. They drank bowl after bowl of the spicy tea which grew on the lower terraces of the conical mountain in better times.

Around midnight they heard the call of the watch fish from the high turrets, "Centipede! Centipede!" They rushed to the highest balcony of the marble palace, where the warrior saw the conical mountain transformed into a monstrous helter-skelter as the centipede spiralled down its sides from the dark lair at the summit, its hundred feet shaking the conical mountain with their incessant tramp, tramp, tramp. And its eyes were vast furnaces of churning liquid heat, burning and flashing. The centipede had grown huge on the lives and the flesh of the Dragon King's kin, its over-gorged maw dribbling the slaver of appetite.

The centipede came closer and closer, its head covering the short patch of ground between the conical mountain and the river lake while its body still spiralled around the mountain, tramp, tramp, tramp. The warrior took his great bow, but reaching into his quiver he found to his dismay that only three arrows remained. He slotted the first arrow into the bow, drew back with a mighty strength, and taking careful aim he let fly. The arrow found its mark, striking the centipede right between the eyes, but bounced off the hard flesh harmlessly. The warrior slotted the second arrow, drawing back with even greater strength. He let fly, and again the arrow found its mark and again it bounced off harmlessly.

Now, the centipede's terrible head had reached the river lake. It towered over the warrior. He felt the burning cauldrons of its eyes as they seared his flesh. He saw the pale, merciless serrations of its teeth. He saw the insatiable, cavernous blackness of its maw. The foul stench of its slimy slaver dribbling from its mouth in torrents made the warrior retch and gag. Then, he remembered. Human spittle is toxic to centipedes.

He drew his last arrow from the quiver and spat upon the arrowhead, "Thwutt!" With slow, immaculate care the warrior slotted the arrow into the bow and shot with all his remaining force.

The arrow found its mark. It burnt steaming into the horny flesh of the centipede's forehead, like acid on human flesh, as the force of the arrow penetrated deep, deep into the centipede's brain. A hundred feet drummed upon the ground.

A hundred segments clashed together like cymbals. The eyes boiled and burnt and flamed like twin volcanoes. Then, their light faded. Silence came. A full moon rose, its pale orb shining on the long bridge and the broken terraces of the conical mountain and reflecting in the dark, quiet waters of the river lake.

The rest of the night was spent in feasting and rejoicing. In the morning, the Dragon King offered the warrior two gifts in thanks for slaying his enemy. The first gift, a bronze bell with a deep, clear tone, the warrior mounted at the centre of his village. To this very day, the tolling of the bell offers perpetual prayers to the warrior's master, the sun god. The second gift was a simple bag of rice. But it was no ordinary bag of rice, for however much the warrior took from it to feed himself and his family, the bag was always full to overflowing.

And so, the warrior became famous throughout the land and was known to all as 'My Lord, Bag of Rice.'

Source

My Lord Bag of Rice is based on the traditional story of the same name, which I found in *The Japanese Fairy Book*, rendered into English by Yei Theodora Osaki, 1903, published by Constable and Company Limited.

Our Psychological Reflection

My Lord Bag of Rice is about having the will to serve a higher cause and the courage to see it through.

This Hawk depicted on the book's cover symbolises the Transpersonal Journey of Soul, the essence of the Transpersonal Journey, distilled into 14 words inviting reflection:

Wind beneath its wings.
Intent on touching the stars,
Hawk's eyes scan the earth.

The wind beneath our wings carries us on a journey, our Journey of Soul.

At each step in our journey, we step into the unknown, remaining intent on touching the stars, whilst our eyes scan the earth. There is no dichotomy; to make our journey, we need to retain our intent whilst we remain grounded. We need to take courage to face whatever comes whilst remaining undaunted. As does the warrior. We are warriors.

We are repeatedly called to take courage. It takes courage to leave the family of origin and take the step into a survival self. It takes courage, with growing self awareness, to seize our independence and start taking our own life decisions. It takes courage to relinquish our egotism and acknowledge we are a part of the whole. It's no wonder we endure life crises.

I regard the Transpersonal self being faced by particular challenges:

Having self-esteem without regressing into hubris.

Expressing our point of view with integrity whilst being willing to listen and seek to understand another's point of view.

Recognising another's right to their point of view, without asserting a counter-argument, yet being willing to engage openly with them towards a synthesis of your differing points of view.

Being responsible for one's own thoughts and feelings, whilst not taking responsibility for another's thoughts and feelings. In the 1958 western film *The Big Country*, the hero, played by Gregory Peck, responds to his fiancé's concern about what other people think by saying, "I'm not responsible for what people think, only for what I am."

In relationships, neither to be dependent nor to put expectation on the other, which means being willing to say what you would like without expectation of receiving it, whilst hearing what the other would like without any obligation to comply. Such differentiation and clarity can be of service to achieving intimacy.

The Young Man, the Lion, and the Yellow-Flowered Storm-Cloud Tree

> *I first told 'The Young Man, the Lion, and the Yellow-Flowered Storm-Cloud Tree' during a storytelling group in the yurt at St Ethelburga's Centre for Reconciliation and Peace, Bishopsgate. Someone videoed it and posted it on YouTube. Maybe you can still find it on YouTube by searching for "The Young Man, the Lion, and the Yellow-Flowered Storm-Cloud Tree".*

As everything begins in the imagination,
healing begins in the imagination.

Synopsis

This is another story about connection with another species. A young man out hunting feels tired and lies down to rest beside a waterhole that is visited by a thirsty lion. The lion keeps the young man to eat later, pushing him into the branches of a yellow flowered storm-cloud tree. When he sees the young man weeping with fear, the thirsty lion licks the tears from his cheeks, then turns to the water hole, a chance for the young man to run away, calling for help. When the villagers are unable to kill the lion, a wise old man offers an ineluctable outcome that is respectful to man and beast.

The Story

One day a young man went hunting; well, he was supposed to be hunting, but he felt tired and lay down to rest beside a waterhole. A short time later, a lion arrived at the waterhole. The lion was very thirsty. When the lion saw the man lying there as if dead, he thought to himself,

"Mm! I realise I'm hungry as well as thirsty. This will do for later."

The young man knew the lion was there. He went into fight/flight mode. as we animals do; he couldn't fight the lion, and he wasn't fast enough to run away, so he did the third thing; he froze and played dead. The lion thought to himself,

"I'd better quench my thirst before I eat this tasty morsel," so he picked the man up and thrust him into the branches of a yellow flowered storm-cloud tree that grew close to the waterhole. The lion turned towards the waterhole, but as he did so he noticed the man's head move a little.

"Well," thought the lion, "that's a bit odd, I thought he was dead," so he went back to the yellow-flowered storm-cloud tree and pushed the man more firmly into its branches. When the young man began to weep, copious tears running down his cheeks, the lion, who was very thirsty by this time, licked the tears from the young man's cheeks. The lion turned back to the waterhole and continued quenching his thirst. With the lion's back turned, the man leapt from the yellow-flowered storm-cloud tree and began to run away. He didn't want to run towards the village, for fear the lion would run after him and attack the village, so he shouted towards some villagers,

"Help me! Help me! I'm being chased by a lion who has carried me and licked tears from my cheeks."

The villagers were alarmed, and anxious for this young man of their village? They wrapped him in hartebeest skins to disguise his spoor and hid him in some bushes, not wanting this young man of their village to be eaten by a lion.

At the entrance to the village there stood a wise old man, who called out a warning,

"A lion is coming, a lion is coming, a lion who has carried the young man and licked tears from his cheeks."

The lion entered the village and began a rampage looking for the young man. In her distress, the mother of the young man screamed out to the men of the village,

"Shoot the lion, shoot the lion before it finds and kills my beloved son."

The men of the village shot their arrows at the lion, but the arrows just glanced off. The men of the village threw their spears at the lion, but the spears just glanced off. The wise old man cautioned the men,

"You cannot kill the lion, for he has carried the young man and licked the tears from his cheeks, and his will is set on his mother's beloved son."

The people of the village offered other children to the lion, but the lion's will was set on the mother's beloved son. The wise old man spoke to the people,

"The mother must give up her beloved son to the lion, for he has carried him and licked the tears from his cheeks and our spears and arrows cannot touch him."

With a heavy heart, the mother of the young man spoke to the men of the village,

"Let it be so, but let not the lion carry my beloved son to his eating place. Let the lion and my son lie in death together."

The villagers unwrapped the young man from the hartebeest skins. They gave him to the lion. The lion killed the young man. The men of the village rushed forward and plunged their spears into the lion. As he was dying, the lion spoke,

"Now I can die. I have been given the young man whom I lifted and carried to the yellow flowered storm-cloud tree. I put him there and licked his tears. I sought him all this time. Now I shall lie with him in peace, for he is mine and I am his."

Sources

Spirit of Trees website, *The Young Man, The Lion, and The Yellow-Flowered Zwart-Storm Tree*, https://spiritoftrees.org/the-young-man-the-lion; Alida Gersie, 1992, from *Earthtales, Storytelling in Times of Change.*

As well as the story, the Spirit of Trees website provides a spiritual commentary on the story.

Search on YouTube—The Young Man, the Lion, and the Yellow-Flowered Storm-Cloud Tree—for my first telling of this tale.

Our Psychological Reflection

The Young Man, the Lion, and the Yellow-Flowered Storm-Cloud Tree brings us full circle, back to *Dream Dilemma*, but with a very different take on our union with the natural world, in the way the story challenges our mindset about our relationship with dangerous predators with whom we share the world.

Bibliography

Callimachus *Erysichthon and the Grove of Demeter*. This is an ancient Greek myth told by Callimachus in ancient times.

Gersie, Alida (1992) *Earthtales, Storytelling in Times of Change*, Green Print.

Macy, Joanna and Brown, Molly Young (2014) *Coming Back to Life: The Updated Guide to the Work That Reconnects*, New Society Publishers.

Osaki, Yei Theodora (Translator) (1903) *The Japanese Fairy Book*, Constable and Company.

Reid, Pippa and Reid, Rachel (Illustrator) (Undated pamphlet) *The Music and Story Experience with Pippa Reid.*

Shankaracharya (1946, 1974), Swami Nikhilananda (Translator) (1974) *Ātmabodha, Meaning Self-Knowledge*, Ramakrishna Vedanta Centre.

Tales of Soul Room

Tales of Soul is a set of stories with a distinct psychological context, tales of mind, heart, and soul, including three explicitly psychological stories that I included in my MA thesis, which was a reflection on the relationship between traditional stories and psychological sufferings.

> *As we develop and grow through life, we deepen Soul.*
>
> *'Vasilisa and Baba Yaga' and 'The Horse of Power' are about healing and redemption. In 'Sir Gawain and the Loathly Lady', the protagonists are mutually redemptive, and the character of Lady Ragnell is a feminist icon.*
>
> *The last three traditional stories in this Room, taken from my thesis 'Telling Tales' for my Psychosynthesis Psychotherapy MA degree, reflect on psychological traumas of childhood.*

DOI: 10.4324/9781003712329-11

Vasilisa and Baba Yaga

Suitable to tell or read to older children

'Vasilisa and Baba Yaga' is a story with the power to heal, to deepen, for teller and listeners, the experience of being a Soul.

I have a principle about traditional tales: I never offer an interpretation, because every listener is free to take what they need from a story. This is particularly true of 'Vasilisa and Baba Yaga'. I sometimes tell the 'Vasilisa and Baba Yaga' story to a group as a form of guided meditation, the story alone having the power to resonate with each participant's individual need for healing.

Let the story tell the story.
The story enables the listener to generate a new way of experiencing themselves, which at the outset is unknown.

Synopsis

As she lay dying, a young mother gives her daughter Vasilisa a parting gift, her blessing, and a wooden doll attired like Vasilisa, telling her, "Whenever you are in trouble, the doll will help you."

After her mother died, Vasilisa finds herself in the power of a cruel stepmother and jealous stepsisters, who make her do all the work. One day, they let the fire go out and send Vasilisa out into the forest to beg fire from Baba Yaga. Fearful of the dark forest, with the help of the doll Vasilisa finds her way to Baba Yaga's compound, surrounded by flaming skulls. As she enters the compound, trembling with fear, Baba Yaga sweeps down in her chariot, a fearsome sight, yet Vasilisa does not flinch from telling Baba Yaga, she has come to beg for fire. Baba Yaga promises that if Vasilisa does all the work for her and completes all other tasks she will be given, she will give her fire. Vasilisa does all the work and with the help of the doll completes the tasks. When Baba Yaga asks how she is able to finish all your tasks, Vasilisa replies, "By the blessing of my mother," which drives Baba Yaga into a fearful rage, "We need no blessings here." She thrusts into Vasilisa's hands a flaming skull on a stick and tells her to be gone. Vasilisa flees through the dark forest, the flaming skull lighting her way home, where the cruel stepmother and jealous stepsisters share a fitting end.

The Story

I have included the title of each scene used in the Vasilisa meditation.

Mother's Deathbed: The Blessing

In a Tzardom far away, a young mother lay dying. Beside her bed there knelt her husband and her daughter Vasilisa. Vasilisa was wearing a black smock and a white blouse embroidered by her mother in all the colours of the rainbow and all the colours in between.

The mother leant towards Vasilisa. She took a wooden doll from under her sheets. It wore a black smock and a white blouse embroidered in all the colours of the rainbow and all the colours in between. The mother handed the doll to Vasilisa.

"This is my parting gift to you, my dear daughter, given to me by my own mother," she said in a faint voice, "My blessing! Whenever you are in trouble, the doll will help you. Feed her when she hungers and give her water when she thirsts. Keep her with you always. But, do not tell a soul about her." Vasilisa put the doll deep into the pocket of her smock.

With that, the mother breathed her last breath. Her soul flew from her like a white bird, soared out of the window, and was gone.

Living with Stepmother

Vasilisa grieved for her mother for many lonely nights. Her father grieved also, but like land lying fallow for a spell, new shoots began to spring up. He married a handsome widow with two lovely daughters. He saw only that these three were well mannered, elegant and refined. But if you were to gaze at them, then close your eyes, on the back of your eyelids you would see the image of rats.

Vasilisa's stepmother and stepsisters plagued and bullied her. They made her fetch and chop wood, rake out and make the fire in the stove, wash the clothes, sweep the yard, cook the food and wait upon them. They hoped Vasilisa would grow thin and rough skinned from her toil, for they were jealous of her beauty and hated her for her gentle nature. All the while they spent their time in idleness, preening and pampering themselves.

Vasilisa did all she was made to do without complaining, even though she was often hungry and tired. She was always helpful and kind towards her stepmother and stepsisters. And all the time Vasilisa grew more lovely, with full breasts and rounded hips and a face as bright as a ripe apple, whilst her stepsisters were narrow chested and their lovely faced were marred by spite. This only made them hate Vasilisa all the more, and they plotted to be rid of her.

"I know," said the stepmother one day, "We shall let the fire in the lanterns go out. Then we shall send Vasilisa to Baba Yaga to beg for fire. Baba Yaga will surely kill her and eat her." And they squealed with delight like rats in offal.

When Vasilisa came home from gathering wood in the forest, she found the house in darkness.

"Step-mother," she said, "We have no fire to light the house and cook the food. What shall we do?"

"You know the forest from gathering wood. You must go and fetch fire. You must beg for fire from Baba Yaga. Go!"

With that, the stepmother gave Vasilisa a stale loaf and a flask of water and turned her out into the dark forest to seek fire from Baba Yaga.

Life in the Forest: The White, Red and Black Riders

Vasilisa felt very frightened. In the distance, wolves howled and bears growled, and even the dry sticks snapping beneath her feet made her tremble with shock. She was alone at night in the deep, dark forest and did not know the way to go to find Baba Yaga. Then she remembered the wooden doll which her mother had given to her, her mother's blessing. She put her hand into the deep pocket of her smock, and there she was. She took out the doll and gave her some water and dry bread. She told the doll of her plight and asked for her help. As Vasilisa made her way through the dark forest, the doll guided her path.

Vasilisa walked all night, guided by her doll. Suddenly, a man dressed in white on a white horse came trotting by. Not long after it was dawn. A short time later, a man dressed in red on a red horse came cantering by. Soon after the sun rose. Vasilisa walked for many hours. Then, a man dressed in black on a black horse came galloping by. Swiftly, it was night.

Vasilisa journeyed many days and nights, and many times the horsemen in white and red and black came trotting and cantering and galloping by. One day Vasilisa came to a compound in the heart of the forest. Its fence was made of dead men's bones. The latches on the gate were bony fingers. On every stake a human skull gazed out into the forest. Vasilisa wondered if this were Baba Yaga's dwelling. The doll told her it was. At that moment, the horseman dressed in black on his black horse galloped by. Black horse and rider leapt the fence and were lost to sight, for swiftly it was night. A moment later and all the skulls blazed with an inner fire, lighting the compound like day.

Living with Baba Yaga: The Tasks

Trembling with fear and clutching her doll deep in the pocket of her smock, Vasilisa lifted the bony latch and entered the compound. There she saw Baba Yaga's hut. It stood on huge, yellow, scaly chicken legs. Sometimes it strolled about the compound. Sometimes it whirled around like a dervish. But always its doorway faced the deepest, darkest part of the forest.

There came a sound like wind roaring through the forest. The great trees shook and creaked; their branches cracked; Baba Yaga descended into the compound in her chariot, a massive mortar which she propelled with a great pestle. As she rode through the forest and across the sky she swept the tracks behind her with a besom made of dead men's hair.

Baba Yaga was a fearsome sight. Her long black hair was wild, all knotted and greasy. Her face was a mass of warts, her eyes a piercing black. Her long nose hooked downwards like a scimitar and her chin hooked upwards towards it like an old crescent moon. All the time, at the end of her narrow nostrils, there lingered a bubble of snot. Over the centuries a stalagmite of snot had formed upon the end of her chin and a stalactite of snot upon the end of her nose, so that the two now almost met.

Baba Yaga's nose twitched,

"I smell Russian bones. Show yourself!" Vasilisa stepped forward.

"Have you come of your own free will, girl, or have you been sent?" croaked Baba Yaga. Her voice trembling, Vasilisa replied,

"Largely of my own free will and twice as much because my step-mother and step-sisters sent me. I come to beg for fire."

Baba Yaga sneered,

"Yes, I know all about you and your step-mother and step-sisters. What makes you think I shall give you fire?"

Clutching her doll, deep in her smock's pocket, Vasilisa replied,

"Because I ask it, Babushka."

"You answer wisely," said Baba Yaga with a hiss, "Otherwise, I should have killed you and gobbled you up." Baba Yaga gave a crooked grin. Vasilisa saw her iron teeth, each one filed sharp as a dagger.

"If I am to give you fire, you must work to pay for it," said Baba Yaga, "Fetch and chop my wood, rake out and make my fire in the stove, wash my clothes, sweep my yard, cook my food and wait upon me. If you do everything I ask, I will give you fire. Otherwise …" As Baba Yaga's lips curled in her crooked grin, her burnished teeth flashed in the light from the skulls and for a moment her eyes too burned with fire, "I shall kill you and gobble you up."

"Now," said Baba Yaga, "Fetch me what is cooking on the stove." It was a hot, thick, dark stew, enough for a dozen full-grown working men. But with a mighty slurping and slopping she supped the lot, leaving only a small cupful for Vasilisa. Then Baba Yaga leapt into her mortar, grasped her pestle and took off into the night sky. And the strange thing was, wherever she appeared in the sky she was always framed against the moon, with her hooked nose and crooked chin, her wild, greasy hair streaming behind her.

She returned in the morning and gave Vasilisa her instructions,

"Gather my wood, make my fire, wash my clothes, sweep my yard, cook my food and wait upon me. And one more thing. Take the wheat from my storehouse and separate the good grain from the mildewed grain. If all this work is not done by morning," said Baba Yaga with a steely grimace, "I will kill you and gobble you up." Then she went into her hut to sleep and later to eat.

When she had finished all the other tasks, Vasilisa began to separate the good grain from the mildewed grain, but the work was very slow and hardly anything had been done before night fell and the skulls burst into flame and Baba Yaga took to the skies.

Vasilisa took out her doll, gave her a little of Baba Yaga's stew, and asked her,

"How shall I ever finish this on time, before Baba Yaga kills me and gobbles me up?"

"Sleep now," whispered the doll, "Morning is wiser than evening." Vasilisa slept. After the white horseman had trotted by and the dawning forest began to stir, the doll gathered together all the birds of the forest and set them to work sifting the corn. When Vasilisa awoke, to her joy and relief there were two piles of wheat in the compound, one good grain and the other mildewed.

At that moment, Baba Yaga returned with a whoosh. When she saw the separate piles of good and mildewed grain, she was secretly pleased, but she hissed,

"You have done well." Then she cried, "My loyal servants and bosom friends, come and grind my wheat." Three pairs of hands appeared in the air and ground the good grains so quickly that the forest air blew white with chaff. When the flour was stored the hands disappeared.

Then Baba Yaga gave Vasilisa her instructions,

"Gather my wood, make my fire, wash my clothes, sweep my yard, cook my food and wait upon me. And one more thing. The poppy seeds in this pot have earth mixed in with them. Wash them one by one. If all this work is not done by the morning," said Baba Yaga, "I will kill you and gobble you up." Then she went into her hut to sleep and later to eat.

When she had finished all the other tasks, Vasilisa began to wash the poppy seeds, but the work was very slow, and almost nothing had been done before Baba Yaga took to the skies.

Vasilisa took out her doll, gave her a little stew, and asked her,

"How shall I ever finish this on time, before Baba Yaga kills me and gobbles me up?"

"Sleep now," whispered the doll, "Morning is wiser than evening." Vasilisa slept. After the white horseman had trotted by and the dawning forest began to stir, the doll gathered together all the mice in the forest and set them to work washing the poppy seeds. When Vasilisa awoke, to her joy and relief there was a pot of clean poppy seeds.

At that moment, Baba Yaga landed in the compound. When she saw the pot of clean poppy seeds, she was secretly pleased, but she hissed,

"You have done well." Then she cried, "My loyal servants and bosom friends, come and press my oil." Three pairs of hands appeared in the air and pressed the oil out into jars so quickly the forest was filled with its fragrance. When the work was done the hands disappeared.

Being Given the Fire: Vasilisa's Questions

Baba Yaga went into her hut and slept. Later, when she sat down to eat, Vasilisa stood nearby with a thoughtful look.

"Well, child," asked Baba Yaga, "What do you have to say?"

"I should like to ask you some questions," replied Vasilisa.

"Ask your questions," said Baba Yaga, "But remember, not every question leads to good. If you know too much you will grow old too soon."

"Thank you, Babushka. Who is the rider in white riding a white horse?"

"Ah! He is my dawning day, my bright dawn."

"And, who is the rider in red riding a red horse?"

"Ah! He is my rising sun, my red sun."

"And who is the rider in black riding a black horse?"

"Ah! He is my dark, black night."

Vasilisa thought to ask about the three pairs of hands, but she saw the hungry look in Baba Yaga's eyes and stayed silent.

"Well, child," crooned Baba Yaga, "Surely you have more questions?"

"No, Babushka. As you said, not every question leads to good. If I know too much I shall grow old too soon."

"You answer wisely," hissed Baba Yaga, "More wisely than your years. How so? And how are you able to finish all your tasks?"

"By the blessing of my mother," replied Vasilisa.

"Blessing!" screamed Baba Yaga. She grew to a towering height. Her massive body shook with rage. Her eyes burnt like the bellowing of hot coals. "Blessing!" she bellowed, "We need no blessings here. They hurt my bones."

With that, she took from the fence a skull with eyes of fire, shoved it on a stick and thrust it into Vasilisa's hand.

"Here's the fire you were sent for. Now, be gone!"

Returning Through the Forest: The Flaming Skull

Vasilisa took the flaming skull, ran from the compound and fled into the forest. The skull lit her path, yet she feared this strange lantern and almost cast it away. As she ran, the man dressed in white on a white horse came trotting by, and the glowing eyes began to flicker and fade with the dawn. A short time later, the man dressed in red on a red horse came cantering by, and the glowing eyes were extinguished with the rising sun. All day she ran, until the man dressed in black on a black horse came galloping by, and with the coming of night the skull's flame rekindled. The skull's glowing eyes, lighting her way, now reassured her.

With the dawn, Vasilisa continued her journey through the forest. The stepmother and stepsisters thought Baba Yaga had killed her and gobbled her up. They saw the eerie light and watched it bobbing through the forest. When they saw Vasilisa they rushed out to meet her.

"We have not been able to have light all the time you have been away," they moaned, "However hard we have tried."

Returning Home: The End of the Journey

And so, Vasilisa returned home triumphant. She had survived. Her dangerous journey was completed. She had come home with fire. But the skull held the stepmother and stepsisters in its steady gaze and bored into them. They could not escape its white heat. The three were burnt to ashes.

Source

Based on the story *Vasilisa the Beautiful* by Aleksandr Afanas'ev. Afanas'ev, Aleksandr and Guterman, Norbert (Translator) (1945) *Russian Fairy Tales*. Pantheon Books. Copyright renewed by Random House (1973).

Vasilisa Meditation

I sometimes tell the *Vasilisa and Baba Yaga* story to a group as a form of guided meditation. First I tell the story to the group. Then, I invite the participants to make themselves comfortable, with cushions and yoga mats, and to close their eyes. I introduce each scene, just using its title, then leave a pause to allow each participant to be free to see the story unfold for themselves in their mind's eye and to notice which scene of the story has the strongest resonance for them. Then we gather in the group for the participants to share their experience of the meditation and say which scene had the strongest resonance: 'I was at my mother's deathbed'; 'I know what it's like being alone in the dark forest'; 'I wanted to cast away the flaming skull, I didn't want the responsibility'.

One woman contacted me beforehand to say that she was unwell and unable to attend. I assured her that the session was simply a meditation based on the story. When I arrived, she was already there, greeting me with a wide grin. When she shared her experience of the meditation, she said, triumphantly,

"I came home with the fire." She tells me later that she had been ill and the Vasilisa meditation had been a turning point in her life.

Reflections

Your Psychological Reflection

For therapeutic storytellers, I invite you to create your own Vasilisa Meditation, suitable for the group with which you work.

Vasilisa and Baba Yaga is a tale with the power to heal. It has the power to heal because anyone who hears the tale may recognise where they are in their own life's journey, and this can help them to move forward. So, I invite you to read the story again slowly, scene by scene, identifying the phases in Vasilisa's Journey of Soulmaking, and asking yourself: where am I in this journey?

Please, reflect on these questions before reading on:

The doll, Vasilisa's mother's parting gift, is something of a puzzle. So, what do you make of this parting gift?

Even more puzzling are the White, Red and Black Riders, what do you make of them?

My Psychological Reflection

Vasilisa and Baba Yaga follows a life's journey: a child at her mother's bedside; a subdued childhood spent with a callous and demanding mother and bullying sisters; her life in the forest, learning to overcome her fears and to move forward; finding a wise-woman whom she can respect and be willing to be guided by, learning to overcome challenges, so as to find the courage to question the wise woman eye to eye. "You answer wisely," responds Baba Yaga, showing Vasilisa that she is ready to receive fire. Returning through the forest, pre-personal doubt assails her before she finds reassurance. Returning home with fire, the vestiges of childhood conditioning are burnt to ashes.

I liken the doll, Vasilisa's mother's parting gift, to Sexuality, the rotating engine driving the expansion of consciousness and will, the active force that directs the development both of consciousness and will throughout life. This is why *Vasilisa and Baba Yaga* makes such an effective meditation; by following Vasilisa's Journey of Soulmaking, participants perceive where they are on their own journey.

Baba Yaga refers to the White, Red and Black Riders as 'my bright dawn, my red sun, my dark, black night', so for me they represent the universal, signifying that Baba Yaga, and now Vasilisa, have gained transpersonal wisdom.

The Horse of Power

Suitable to tell or read to older children

There are many traditional tales about redemption, including some in this Collection, for example, the redemption of Richard Galis by the 'witches' of Windsor in the Beastly Tales Room. Another tale in the present Room, 'Vasilisa and Baba Yaga', is the story of the redemption of Vasilisa by the powerful witch Baba Yaga.

Some traditional tales concern the redemption of the feminine by the masculine or the masculine by the feminine. 'The Horse of Power' is a tale of the redemption of a man, the young archer, by a woman, Princess Vasilisa no less.

I was once booked to tell a tale at the wedding of a Kazakhstani couple, in the company of many Kazakhstani family members, the men wearing traditional felt hats, including the father of the bride. The tale I told was 'The Horse of Power', using my djembe drum to accompany the story, varying the rhythm as the young archer gallops to meet with Princess Vasilisa, through the deep forests, across the great steppes, and over the stony mountains, to the edge of the world, where the red sun rises in flame from behind the blue sea. The bride's sister provided her father with a simultaneous translation. As I finished the story, the father of the bride, who knew this Russian story, beamed with pleasure.

On another occasion, exquisite singer and storyteller Hilary Watkins and I gave a joint performance of 'The Horse of Power' in the yurt at St Ethelburga's Centre for Reconciliation and Peace, Bishopsgate. I told the tale, and Hilary sang extempore songs between scenes. It was wonderful to provide such a performance.

I have included the titles of the scenes within 'The Horse of Power' story.
The right story holds up a mirror to the listener's existential experience,
and it is this which brings healing and transformation.

Synopsis

An impulsive young archer finds a firebird's golden feather as he rides the Horse of Power through the forest. Against the advice of the Horse of Power, "Leave the feather where it lies, else you will rue the day and learn the meaning of fear," the young archer takes the firebird's golden feather to the cruel Tzar in hope of reward. Instead, the young archer learns the meaning of fear.

The Story

Bringing the Firebird's Feather

The forest was utterly still. There was no birdsong in the canopy. No rustling of small mammals in the undergrowth. Just the gentle thump of the great horse's hooves caressing the forest floor. The Horse of Power, untold hands high, unbroken, unshod, without saddle or bridle, the young archer on his back riding with his consent.

On the ground before them, something glinting in a shaft of sunlight, a feather from the firebird's burning breast. The firebird had passed this way, filling the forest with silent awe and fear.

The young archer slipped down from the horse's back, bent to pick up the feather,

"This will be a gift to the Tzar, he will reward me handsomely and take me into his service. No Tzar has a feather from the firebird's breast."

The Horse of Power spoke, "Leave the feather where it lies, else you will rue the day and learn the meaning of fear."

But the young archer, in his eager ambition, took no heed.

They cantered through the forest to the palace, and leaving the Horse of Power in the courtyard the young archer rushed excitedly into the presence of the Tzar, knelt before him and laid the firebird's feather at his feet.

The Tzar's heart filled with pride to possess what no other Tzar possessed, but his mouth curled with greed and malice,

"A feather is not a fit gift for a great Tzar. If you can bring a firebird's feather you can bring the firebird, and I will reward you with silver and gold. Else, by my sword your head will no longer sit between your shoulders. Bring me the bird."

The young archer ran into the courtyard weeping with disappointment and dread and told the Horse of Power what the Tzar had demanded. The horse pawed the ground and shook its great head, and the words hung in the air between them, you will rue the day and learn the meaning of fear.

"Do not fear," said the horse, "the trial is not now, the trial is to come. Now, you have a journey to make."

Bringing the Firebird

Guided by the Horse of Power, the young archer begged the Tzar for a thousand bushels of maize, and journeying to the great field at the heart of the kingdom, he had the maize scattered at midnight upon the ground. Then, he shinned up the mighty oak at the centre of the field, hid himself among its branches, and waited for the dawn.

As the red sun rose from out the eastern lands, a great wind blew up, tearing at the forest canopy, the seas at the edge of the world piling themselves up into mountains of spray and dashing themselves against the distant shores. The firebird flew from out the sun, fiery wings outstretched and breast of gold burning bright. It alighted on the field, folded its wings, and greedily began to eat the maize.

The Horse of Power sauntered around the field, pretending to graze but drawing closer and closer to the firebird, until with a sudden lunge he trapped the firebird's fiery wing beneath his mighty hoof. Shinning down from the oak tree the young archer threw a wide net over the firebird, binding it tight. With the firebird over his shoulder, he staggered bent-backed to the palace to receive his reward, leaving behind him a trail of golden feathers. Entering the presence of the Tzar he flung the firebird at his feet. It filled the Tzar's heart with cruel rapture, for since the beginning of time no Tzar had had a firebird casually cast before him like a brace of pigeons.

The Tzar turned to the young archer, his mouth curling with greed and desire,

"What is a bird after all? If you can get the bird you can get my bride, whom I have awaited for so long, Princess Vasilisa. Bring her, from the edge of the world, where the red sun rises in flame from behind the blue sea, and I will reward you with silver and gold. Else, by my sword, your head will no longer sit between your shoulders. Bring me my bride."

The young archer ran into the courtyard weeping with chagrin and dread, told the Horse of Power what the Tzar had demanded. The horse pawed the ground, shook its great head, and the words hung in the air between them, you will rue the day and learn the meaning of fear.

"Do not fear," said the horse, "the trial is not now, the trial is to come. Now, you have a journey to make."

Bringing Vasilisa

Guided by the Horse of Power, the young archer begged the Tzar for a silver tent with a golden canopy, fine carpets, rich wines, and tasty delicacies, and with these they journeyed. Through the deep forests. Across the great steppes. Over the stony mountains. To the edge of the world, where the red sun rises in flame from behind the blue sea.

Whilst the Horse of Power wandered on the beach, its great hooves sinking into the sand, the young archer raised the silver tent with its golden canopy beside the shore, laid out the fine carpets, wines and delicacies, and began to regale himself of the tasty dishes.

Princess Vasilisa sat lightly in her silver boat, lightly dipping her golden oars in the blue sea, moving the silver boat lightly through the dancing waves, closer and closer to the edge of the world, where she saw the silver tent with its golden canopy and the young archer. Her silver boat crunched against the golden sand, and stepping ashore Princess Vasilisa approached the silver tent and seated herself on a fine carpet beneath the golden canopy. The young archer bowed low and invited her to partake of the rich wines and tasty delicacies. They ate with delight and toasted each other in the rich wine from golden goblets until the Princess' eyelids began to close, the golden goblet fell from her fingers and she lay back on the carpet in a deep sleep. To the young archer, she was the image of loveliness. Quickly, he rolled her in the carpet, laid her gently over the horse's back and set off back to the palace. Over the stony mountains. Across the great steppes. Through the deep forests.

Entering the presence of the Tzar, the young archer unrolled the carpet to reveal the sleeping princess.

"Sound the trumpets," called the Tzar, "Ring the bells. For we are to wed."

The ringing of bells woke Vasilisa,

"Where is my blue sea? Where is my silver boat and my golden oars?"

"The blue sea is far away. For your silver boat I give you a golden throne. The trumpets sound for our wedding. The bells are ringing for our joy."

The princess turned away from the Tzar with his cruel eyes and curled lips, and turned to the young archer with love in her heart for one fit to ride the Horse of Power. Then, she spoke to the Tzar,

"I will not marry without my wedding gown. At the edge of the world, where the red sun rises in flame from behind the blue sea, my wedding gown lies in a golden casket beneath a great stone in the middle of the blue sea."

The Tzar turned to the young archer, his mouth curling with desire and frustration,

"How could you bring my bride without her wedding gown? Bring her gown from the edge of the world, else, by my sword, your head will no longer sit between your shoulders. Bring me the frock."

The young archer ran into the courtyard weeping with anguished love and told the Horse of Power what the Tzar had demanded. The horse pawed the ground and shook its great head, and the words hung in the air between them, you will rue the day and learn the meaning of fear.

"Do not fear," said the horse, "the trial is not now, the trial is to come. Now, you have a journey to make."

Bringing the Wedding Gown

The young archer and the Horse of Power journeyed through the deep forests. Across the great steppes. Over the stony mountains. To the edge of the world, where the red sun rises in flame from behind the blue sea.

The young archer looked sadly at the blue sea. But the Horse of Power searched the shore until he found a great lobster crawling sideways across the golden sand. When the lobster came close, the horse slowly lifted a foreleg and brought the hoof down gently but firmly on the lobster's tail. The lobster struggled in vain against the heavy hoof, then screamed,

"I am the Tzar of all the lobsters. Release me and we shall do whatever you ask."

The horse released the lobster and said what he must do. The Tzar of all the lobsters stood at the edge of the world and called out. The blue sea seemed to boil with white foam and from its depths crawled thousands of lobsters bearing the golden casket, taken from beneath the great stone in the middle of the blue sea. Taking the casket, the young archer thanked the Tzar of all the lobsters, and leaping onto the horse's back they began their journey back to the palace. Over the stony mountains. Across the great steppes. Through the deep forests.

Later, the princess appeared in her wedding gown, lovelier than daylight, more beautiful than the stars of heaven. The Tzar looked at her with hard, hungry eyes and held his hand out to her, but she would not take it,

"I will not marry until the one who brought me here has done penance in boiling water."

His lips curling with ingratitude and malice, the Tzar commanded his servants,

"Make a great fire, set upon it the largest cauldron of water, and when it boils take this creature and cast him into the boiling water to do penance for bringing my bride from the edge of the world."

The young archer's heart was all despair at losing his life at the behest of the woman he had so shortly come to love.

"Great Tzar," he said, "suffer me before I die to bid farewell to my horse."

At a sign from the princess, the Tzar assented,

"But make it quick, for our nuptials await."

The young archer ran into the courtyard weeping in an agony of betrayal and fear, told the Horse of Power what Princess Vasilisa had demanded and the Tzar had ordered, and would have made his farewell. But the horse pawed the ground, shook its great head, and the words hung in the air between them, you will rue the day and learn the meaning of fear.

"The trial is now, the trial is come. Now you have a final journey to make."

The Trial

The horse was secretly encouraged by what Princess Vasilisa had done. All the same, he guided the young archer on how he might face the trial, face death.

The great cauldron was coming up to the boil. Princess Vasilisa remained impassive. The Tzar was torn between his relish to see the young archer's suffering and his desire for the princess. The young archer, standing firmly in the grip of two servants, was full of dread resolution.

The princess stepped towards the cauldron. She moved her hand over the bubbling and seething water. Her lips briefly moved. A fleeting, enigmatic smile flickered across her features,

"The water boils. All is ready."

As the drums rolled, the young archer wrenched himself free of his captors. He ran boldly forward and flung himself into the boiling foam. He swirled around and around, twice sinking below the surface and rising again. He sank for the third and last time. The Tzar's lips curled with malicious pleasure. The princess' face shone with enigmatic glee. And the young archer leapt from the cauldron and stood before them in the full flower of mature manhood.

The Tzar stared at the apparition risen before him, his lips curling with envy and spite. He thought of his own grey hairs, his bent back, gnarled face, and toothless gums,

"If the waters can work this miracle for a mere archer then what can they work for a mighty Tzar?" He stumbled forward and climbed into the cauldron to a terrible death. The servants boiled the flesh from his bones for pig meal and cast the bones to his dogs.

The young man became the new Tzar. The princess became Tzarina. Each loving the other, they ruled wisely and well until the time for the Tzar to journey to the next world and for Vasilisa to follow her next call.

Source

Based on the story *The Firebird and Princess Vasilisa* by Aleksandr Afanas'ev. Afanas'ev, Aleksandr, Guterman, Norbert (Translator) (1945) *Russian Fairy Tales*. Pantheon Books. Copyright renewed by Random House (1973).

Reflections

Your Psychological Reflection

I invite you to make a list of the main characters in the story. How many are they?

For each character, ask yourself:

How do they use their energy? Is their energy stuck, and if so, how?
Soul is their whole, lived experience. How do you imagine their Soul experience to be?
Sexuality is the rotating engine driving the expansion of consciousness and will. What do you discern about their consciousness and will?
Spirit has a capacity to be self-reflective, make choices, exercise will, create change, be self-determined, and present their personality to the world. How would you describe their Spirit?
To what extent have they expanded Spirit and deepened Soul during the story?
How powerful are they? What is the basis of their power?

Which character holds the most power, and why? Which carries the most authority, and why?

What is the journey the young archer really needs to make? Describe the journey.

Which character do you identify with, and why?

My Psychological Reflection

I don't want to spoil your fun, so I shan't provide answers to these questions. Anyway, it's down to you as the reader what you take from the story. So, I shall go off at a tangent.

There is a tale of a young archer, on the slippery slope of addiction and obsession. Young Man falls for the lure of silver and gold, despite Better Judgement.

Then, Young Man can't stop; the craving just gets worse; he wants more; now he wants the trappings of power, even at risk of his life, still despite Better Judgement. When Young Man espies a princess by the golden sands he sees her just as an object to prize, a trophy wife. Then there's Tzar, proud, greedy, malicious, possessive, and controlling. Tzar is obsessed by the princess, desirous of having her as a wife in his cruel power. Tzar is immune to Better Judgement.

When the princess appears in her finest gown, lovelier than daylight, more beautiful than the stars of heaven, she is a real person. She is one who can appeal to Better Judgement, calling out Young Man to be bold, to summon the courage to transform the impulse of craving into the quality of passion. Tzar energy is subsumed. With the alignment of the clear-sighted princess, who sees the young archer and his quality of passion, the young archer comes to stand before her in the full flower of mature manhood.

To my mind, there is only one thing that can overcome addiction, and that is something stronger than the addiction. And the princess has it.

Here's another story about overcoming addiction. Doctor Naseeruddin practises in Bombay. He smokes 60 cigarettes a day. He tells a sick patient that he has to give up smoking. The patient replies, "Doctor, I will if you will." In service of his patient, Doctor Naseeruddin never smokes again. This is a true story; only his name is changed.

Sir Gawain and the Loathly Lady

A tale to be told or read to older children and adults

> *'Sir Gawain and the Loathly Lady' is a humorous Arthurian tale, with a vitally significant contemporary punch, about honouring the rights of women.*
>
> *It is a terrific tale to tell, especially to 9- to 11-year-old children. We cannot start soon enough to acquaint children with the importance of affirming the rights of women.*
>
> *The story has lots of scope for children to express all that nauseating bodily stuff that kids (and me) enjoy so much. For the storyteller, there is a wonderful opportunity for characterisation in voice and mannerism, with such strong protagonists as a querulous king, an honourable but emotionally detached knight, and most of all the loathly lady, the true hero of the story; Lady Ragnell is a feminist icon, and rightly so.*
>
> *When I write the above paragraph about characterisation and strong protagonists, I discover a new depth in the story. In my subsequent redraft, I seek to convey the profound wisdom inherent in the story, whilst acknowledging it as a boisterous tale to tell to older children as well as to adults.*

As everything begins in the imagination,
healing begins in the imagination.

Synopsis

An internet reviewer[1] wrote about Ethel Johnston Phelps' *Gawain and the Lady Ragnell* (see *Source* below) and how Lady Ragnell imagines gaining Gawain's hand in marriage, "The lady must move deliberately by first entrapping King Arthur, then getting Gawain's consent to an unwelcome alliance, and, most difficult of all, making sure that Gawain trusts and respects her enough to let her make the crucial decision."

The Story

King Arthur was visiting Carlisle Castle with Sir Gawain, the finest knight in all the land. It was a sunny day, and King Arthur had an appetite for hunting in Inglewood forest. When he returned, he looked pale and distraught.

"My liege, what has happened," enquired Sir Gawain, for it didn't seem right to see his king in such a state.

The king told his tale,

"I am deep in Inglewood forest, chasing a great white stag. I am unarmed, save for my bow and quiver of arrows. I am distracted—letting the stag escape into the depth of the forest—by the appearance of a tall knight in black armour, sword raised.

'Sir knight,' I appeal to him, 'by the laws of chivalry, you cannot draw sword on an unarmed man.'

The knight sneers,

'I shall not kill you this day, but I shall kill you in a year and a day, unless you can answer a simple question.'

Puzzled, I ask,

'What question can this be?' He answers,

'I am Sir Gromer Somer Joure, and I seek revenge for the loss of my northern lands. The question is this, what does a women most desire, above all else?' I grovel,

'I promise you, sir knight, I shall be here without fail in a year and a day, unarmed, with an answer to your question. Now, please let me depart.'"

Ending his story, the king tells Gawain,

"I find the question quite perplexing, most troubling, so perhaps, Gawain, you can help me search out the answer, so as to save my life."

"What a puzzle, we can have a little fun with this," smiled Gawain, until he saw his lord's face, all forlorn. "Mm!" he mused, "Quite a puzzle."

> *{I say to the listeners, I think Arthur and Gawain need some help here. So, tell me, what's your answer to the question, what does a woman most desire, above all else? I get lots of answers, gold, jewels, chocolate, shoes, a handsome husband.... I'll let Arthur and Gawain know, I say. The tale goes on. }*

"Don't be so downhearted, my liege," says Gawain, confident of success, "Mount up. We'll scour the land to find the answer."

They return a year later, their saddlebags stuffed with answers, but with failing confidence they really have the right answer.

A day before King Arthur must meet Sir Gromer Somer Joure, he wandered off alone. On his way back, Gawain met him on the road,

"My liege, you look somewhat of a pother," and King Arthur began to tell his tale,

"I ride to the edge of the forest, where I encounter a grotesque woman. Her girth is as great as her height. Her face is covered in ...

> *{Actually, you can help me out here, what do you think she looks like? The lurid imagination of children knows no bounds. I find it hilarious. }*

'You have to answer Sir Gromer Somer Joure's question tomorrow,' the woman sneers discourteously at me.

'Humph! Humph! What's it got to do with you?'

In a sing-song voice, she answers,

'Da-da-di-da-da! You don't know the answer.'

'Then, tell me the answer and I'll give you a bag of gold.'

'No use for go-old!'

'A mound of jewels!'

'No use for jew-els!'

'Land aplenty!'

'No use for la-and!'

'You're kidding me, you don't know the answer at all.'

'Ah, but I do. Sir Gromer Somer Joure is my stepbrother. I am the Lady Ragnell, and I know his wicked ways.'

'Humph! Humph! You don't want gold, you don't want jewels, you don't want land. So, what do you want?'"

Ending his tale, Arthur began muttering to himself,

"Loathsome wench, I'll try the other answers first, she shan't have what she wants," until Gawain became exasperated,

"Your talking nonsense, my lord, for goodness sake, you need to tell me what she wants." He gradually wheedles the rest of the tale out of Arthur, eyes cast down, chin on his chest, more chided child than mighty king.

" 'What I want,' the Lady Ragnell pauses, 'is to have the finest knight in all the land, Sir Gawain, as my husband.'

'Humph! Humph! But that's impossible, Gawain's not mine to give away, he's his own man.' 'His own man, yes, I want him to marry me of his own free will.'

'Humph! Humph! Out of the question! I won't even put your proposal to him.'

'Whatever! Maybe you'll change your mind, so I'll wait for you here tomorrow.'"

Arthur ended his tale,

"So, there you have it, Gawain, you can't possibly marry such a repellent woman."

Gawain stalwartly disagreed, with a slight lifting of his chin, saying,

"No problem! I would do anything to save your life, my liege," whilst putting aside the thought of such a spouse. "When the Lady Ragnell's answer has saved your life, then she and I shall wed."

The following day, Arthur rode alone and unarmed to the edge of Inglewood forest, where the Lady Ragnell, with a triumphal smile, gave Arthur the answer he needed. Then, he rode on to his fateful encounter with a jubilant Sir Gromer Somer Joure, whose black armour shone in a shaft of sunlight.

"On your knees, my liege," he sneered, raising high his sword, "So, tell me, what does a women most desire, above all else?"

Arthur tried other answers first,

"Gold!"

"NO-O!"

"Jewels!"

"NO-O!"

"Chocolate!"

"NO-O!"

"Shoes!"

"NO-O!"

"A handsome husband!"

"NO-O!"

Sir Gromer Somer Joure waved his sword menacingly,

"You have failed, prepare to die."

In desperation, Arthur bellowed,

"Wait, I have one more answer, what a woman desires above all else is the right and power to exercise her own will."

For a moment, Sir Gromer Somer Joure stood aghast, then became consumed with anger. Dropping his sword, he raged,

"That loathsome stepsister gave you the answer, that Ragnell, I'll chop off her head, I'll ..."

Uttering abominable oaths—that I couldn't possibly recount here—without once repeating himself, his voice diminishing as he ran deeply into Inglewood forest, he fled.

It was a glum King Arthur and an exultant Lady Ragnell who met Sir Gawain on the road to Carlisle Castle. Arthur whispered to Gawain, suggesting the marriage might be deferred, perhaps indefinitely, but Gawain's response was clear,

"By my oath of chivalry as a knight and my promise to Lady Ragnell, I shall wed the lady today."

News quickly spread that Gawain was to wed the loathly lady, so a large crowd was gathered to greet the three as they entered Carlisle Castle, and to get a good look at Gawain's loathly bride. The wedding was promptly arranged, with 40 bishops and archbishops, including the Archbishop of Canterbury, who performed the ceremony. At the wedding banquet, two benches were set side by side at the top table to accommodate the bride's girth. She laughed boisterously and talked incessantly throughout the meal, drinking and eating copiously, spraying masticated morsels onto the plates of horrified guests, and farting stentoriously. Gawain was courteous and attentive throughout, plying his bride with tasty titbits and keeping her cup of wine filled to the brim. At the close of the wedding feast, bride, and groom were escorted to the bridal chamber. They were at last alone.

Gawain and his bride faced each other. Ragnell, with a quizzical smile, said,

"Well, husband, you have treated me with unfailing courtesy, honour, and respect, and at no time have you shown disgust of my loathly looks. So, now, husband, gimme a kiss. Unflinching, always a gallant knight, Gawain leant forward and lightly kissed her on the lips." Then he jumped back in shock, shrieking,

"What wizardry is this?" For, before him now was a lovely, slender young women, with long black hair, piercing black eyes, and a mischievous smile upon her shapely lips, dressed in a simple, elegant grey gown. Gawain felt unmanned.

Perceiving his discomfiture, she asked an astute question,

"Don't you prefer me like this? Or, would you rather I stayed the loathly lady?"

Gawain was flummoxed,

"No... yes... what... but! Of course I like you like this, but how can it be?"

"My stepbrother, Sir Gromer Somer Joure, has always hated me. He sought control of me and all I possess. When I defied him, he accused me of being unwomanly. His mother being skilled in wizardry, he used her magic to turn me into the loathly lady you met earlier. I couldn't regain my true shape until the greatest knight in all the land, loathsome as I was, were to marry me of his own free will. Through your faithfulness, you have achieved the unachievable."

His voice cracking as his unfamiliar tears overflowed, Gawain uttered,

"My sweet love, now the evil spell is broken."

"Only partly so, my love," was her tender reply, "for you have to make a choice. I can only be as I am now for half the day, and for the other half I must be the loathly lady. This is your choice; I can be lovely by day and loathly by night or loathly by day and lovely by night. If I am lovely by day, the whole court will admire and envy you. If I am loathly by day, the whole court will deride and ridicule you. The nights? They speak for themselves. What is your choice?"

Without hesitation, Gawain knelt before her,

"Madam, I cannot make that choice for you, for it is a choice about your own self, which you need to make of your own free will."

She clasped him in her arms, their tears flowing together,

"My dearest love, you have answered truly, affirming what I desire as a woman above all else, the right and power to exercise my own will, and in this the wicked spell is fully broken."

And so, in love, joy, tears, and rejoicing, commenced the marriage of Sir Gawain and the Lady Ragnell.

Source

The story *Gawain and the Lady Ragnell* appears in Ethel Johnston Phelps' book *The Maid of the North: Feminist Folk Tales from Around the World.*

Reflections

Egalitarian Reflection

The Lady Ragnell is a feminist icon. What does 'the Lady Ragnell is a feminist icon' really mean for you?

Your Psychological Reflection

What impression does this story leave with you?

The main characters are King Arthur, Sir Gromer Somer Joure, Sir Gawain, and the Lady Ragnell. For each character:

What is your assessment of their psychological development?

Where is their centre of gravity?

What development takes place during the story?

Which character do you most identify with, and why?

My Psychological Reflection

A recurring theme in traditional tales is the redemption of the feminine by the masculine or the masculine by the feminine. In this story it's both. Lady Ragnell is not only the hero of this story, but she is also instrumental in humanising Gawain, redeeming him from his emotional detachment.

The psychological context of *Sir Gawain and the Loathly Lady* is redemption discovered through relationship. As Schwartz-Salant (1998) writes, "Rarely, if ever, can a person enter the path of creating and transforming a self without the fire and challenge of an ongoing relationship."

There is no lack of fire and challenge in the relationship between Sir Gawain and the Loathly Lady, her eating, drinking, and farting habits for starters. In spite of such provocation, Gawain remains courteous and attentive, and as the lady remarks, calling him 'husband', he treats with unflinching courtesy, honour, and respect the woman with whom he has chosen to enter into wedlock. He does so because he had done so. Likewise the lady, acting toward Gawain with such sweet, loving, and gentle humour as to draw from him unfamiliar tears. When, without sway, she offers him a choice, without hesitation he responds with a third choice: it is a choice about your own self, which you needs to make of your own free will.

To my mind, theirs is a transpersonal marriage. They treat each other with courtesy and respect. There is no ego projection or personal assertion. So, their marriage commences in love, joy, tears, rejoicing, and freedom.

Telling Tales

My incomparable and insightful thesis tutor Roger Evans, responding to the penultimate version of my MA thesis 'Telling Tales', whilst assuring me the thesis would pass, suggested I reflect on one particular paragraph. My reflection on the three main phases of human development, pre-personal, personal, and transpersonal, yielded the essence of psychospiritual development in three sentences:

Ego is built through mirroring.
Personal self is attained through self-reflection.
Self is realised by the individual seeing through to the universal.

I wrote the tales collected in this book over a long period, without thought for any underlying psychological meaning. This book's purpose has been to explicate this meaning without changing a single word in the stories themselves.

The following three tales are an exception. I recognised the way traditional stories can so sharply convey the vicissitudes of a 'wounded child' as they may present in therapy, selected these three tales as illustration, then wrote my versions to include in my MA thesis. This means I can sail closer to the interpretational wind than anywhere else in this book.

'Telling Tales' draws on Stephen Johnson's (1994) use of descriptive names—The Owned Child, The Hated Child, The Abandoned Child—to illustrate the character styles portrayed in the next three stories:

'The Feeling In Her Bones' is the story of The Owned Child, whose life issue is to gain a clear sense of their own identity. The story portrays a child whose controlling father divests her of any sense of her own identity.

'The Juniper Tree' is the story of The Hated Child, whose life issue is to feel safe and secure in the presence of others. The story portrays a child whose mother cannot provide the secure loving care, devotion, and attention he needs for his wellbeing.

'Saint Corentin and the Golden Fish' is the story of The Abandoned Child, whose life issue is to have their emotional needs met. The story portrays a child whose mother can provide his need for a place to live and for food and clothing, but she cannot meet his emotional needs. In this story, the abandoned child, as a grown man, now faces the inevitable mid-life crisis

The story is the healer.

Your Psychological Reflection

For the next three *Telling Tales* stories, I invite you to reflect on the stories and my egalitarian and psychological reflections in the light of your own experience of owned, hated, and abandoned 'children' in your therapy room.

The Feeling In Her Bones

'The Feeling In Her Bones' is the story of The Owned Child. It is a story of abuse, transformation, and the restoration of a lost soul.

The first story I ever told to a live audience was on my storytelling course at Bleddfa in Radnorshire. In the afternoon, I was trying to prepare a story from CP Estes' literally wonderful book 'Women Who Run with the Wolves', except that I repeatedly flipped over to a different story in the same book, 'Skeleton Woman'.

Eventually, I realised that Skeleton Woman wanted her story to be heard, so this was the first story I ever told to a live audience.

In the evening at Bleddfa, we storytelling students had the opportunity to tell tales to an audience of local people and holidaymakers, led by the phenomenal storyteller Duncan Williamson, a Scottish traveller and Pict with a fund of 3,000 stories, any of which he could tell at the drop of a hat.

I was told later by a woman student that as I spoke the phrase 'with the rhythm of the waves, the rhythm of the tides', Duncan was mouthing the phrase with me. As I finished the story, Duncan rose, pointed at me, and said to the audience,

"This is a brilliant storyteller."

As a fledgling storyteller, I felt moved and affirmed.

The story is the healer
and serves as a container for each listener's Soul energy.

Synopsis

A young woman is thrown over a cliff into the sea by her father. Lying on the seabed, her flesh is eaten by fish, and only her bones and the feeling in her bones remain. One day, a sailor fishes her out at the end of his line, and aghast at the sight flees in fear for his home. But the woman, being caught up in his line, follows him home. He's in for a shock and gets more than he realised.

The Story

Afterwards, no-one could remember what had caused the violent rift between father and daughter. But a rift there was, and now the father stands at the top of the hill, above the sheer cliffs, above the small bay, with the young woman struggling weakly in his arms. Her heavy, heavy heart is all despair.

He flings her over the cliff. She falls, down, down into the water. Because her heart is heavy, she sinks down, down to the bottom of the sea. For a moment, before she sinks into unconsciousness, she feels the desolation in her heart.

As she lies at the bottom of the sea, her honey flesh turns grey. Crabs crawl over her and sink their pincers into her flesh. Great fishes feast upon her. She is picked clean. Her golden hair drifts away upon the tide.

She is without sight or hearing, taste or smell, without touch, and without memory. All that is left is the feeling in her bones, which serve for sight and senses. And where her heart once was, there is a heavy, heavy hollow. Time passes. She adapts to the rhythm of the waves, forever rocking backwards and forwards, the rhythm of the tide, forever shifting this way and that over the shingle.

Fishermen no longer come to this bay, at first out of respect, later out of fear, for it came to be thought a haunted place. Many ages pass. Until one day a fisherman braver than the rest ventures into the bay despite the dire warnings of the other fishermen. There is an edge of apprehension in him as he paddles into the bay and as he feeds his line over the pulley in the stern of the boat.

He casts his line, and it goes down, down to the very bottom, where it becomes entangled in the woman's ribcage. The line tightens as she shifts across the shingle, and the fisherman heaves and heaves, imagining some great salmon or bream impaled upon his hook. But the hollow where her heart once was is heavier than he. Then, with the unfamiliar tugging of the line, she is for a moment distracted from the heaviness where her heart once was, and in that moment she rockets out of the sea and jams her fingers in the pulley.

The fisherman falls back into the bottom of the boat and stares aghast at the apparition which has risen before him, her hand raised. In terror he grabs the paddle and paddles for the shore as fast as he can, glancing over his shoulder as he goes. But the faster he goes the faster she follows, and the faster she follows the faster he goes. His heart is hammering against his rib cage. His blood scorches through his veins like summer fire. But he does not escape her.

As the boat crunches hard against the shore her fingers come loose from the pulley, and she falls, a heap of bones, into the boat. At the same moment, grabbing his precious line, the fisherman leaps for the shore and pounds and scrambles and tears across the sand and rocks and fields and hedges and ditches towards his hut. But all the time he hears her behind him, crunching over the sand, scraping over the rocks, and rattling over the fields. The hut gets nearer, its heavy oak door standing open. Heart hammering, blood scorching, he throws himself into the hut, slamming and bolting the door in a single movement, and falling thankfully onto the hard earth floor.

Time passes. His heart slows. His blood cools. He scrabbles around in the dark for tinder and flint to light the lamp. As the warm light reaches out to fill the hut, "Aah!" She leans against the door post, staring at him through the sockets of her eyes. He cowers in a corner in terror, as far from her as possible, but cannot escape those staring eyes. They stare at one another. Time passes. She has not moved nor done him harm. His terror is slowly overcome by curiosity. He creeps warily over to where she lies. He sees his line entangled in her ribcage. With understanding, his fear gives way to waves of relief. Crouching over her, he looks at her for some time, a tangle of bones. An unfamiliar feeling flutters in his heart, and with compassion he gently disentangles the line from her ribcage and tenderly straightens out her bones.

Exhausted by terror and exertion, he sinks onto a pile of rugs, draws a thick blanket over himself and falls into a deep sleep. With the feeling in her bones, the woman knows the rhythm of the waves, the rhythm of the tide. Rocking and shifting with the rhythm of the waves, the rhythm of the tide, she moves herself slowly over to where the fisherman lies. She creeps over the rugs and under the blanket, wrapping her bony arms around his chest and her bony legs around his thighs.

The fisherman is a lonely man. As he dreams of his loneliness, first one tear then another trickles down his cheek. The tears evoke in her feelings of thirst and then hunger. She knows in her bones that she is—*{what?}*—undernourished! Laughter brings her fresh heart, where the heavy hollow had been. She sips the tears from his cheek. As the tears nourish her new flesh forms around her bones.

First, lips and tongue to sip the tears, a throat to swallow, a stomach to absorb; breasts and belly, back and buttocks; a soft creek between her legs; until at last she is made whole. Meanwhile the fisherman has been dreaming of a wife, with golden hair, honey flesh, firm breasts, and a soft creek between her legs. And in the morning when he wakes he finds himself entangled in the arms and legs of the wife of his dreams, with golden hair, honey flesh, firm breasts, and a soft creek between her legs.

Sources

The story is loosely based on the story *Skeleton Woman* by Clarissa Pinkola Estés (1992); The Story Museum, www.storymuseum.org.uk/1001-stories/skeleton-woman.

Reflections

Egalitarian Reflection

My point, in relating how I told the story at Bleddfa, is that Duncan appreciated the story's meaning in a way that I failed to do until later, and in particular he knew that the phrase 'with the rhythm of the waves, the rhythm of the tides' is the turning point of the story. Up to this point in the story, the woman had been a helpless victim, under the control of father, crabs, fish, waves, tides, and even the fisherman as he hauled her out of the sea. The phrase 'with the rhythm of the waves, the rhythm of the tides' marks the moment when the woman begins to assert her own will and to realise her own future.

Later, one of the women students, possibly mindful of hurt she had herself suffered, says to me,

"I am so glad you included the part where the father threw his daughter into the sea." Like Duncan, she too had understood the true meaning and depth of the story, as I then began to do.

My Psychological Reflection

The Feeling In Her Bones is the psychological story of The Owned Child. It is another story about redemption discovered through relationship, and the turning point in the story is the turning point for the woman, when she begins to assert her personal will.

The Story Museum lists *Skeleton Woman* as an Inuit story, retold and highly popularised, by Dr CP Estes. The Story Museum tells us that this is 'a folk tale for older children and teenagers'. I demur. Teenagers, maybe, but I view this as an adult story about fathers' abuse of their daughters—or more generally, men's abuse of women. When I wrote my own version of the story, *The Feeling In Her Bones*, I did so from this perspective.

My telling of this tale to an anonymous client is included in the *Storytelling as a Healing Art* section.

The Juniper Tree

> *This is a horror story. A powerful, complex, psychological story. A story of The Hated Child.*
>
> *The meaning of the story is in its name, 'The Juniper Tree'; the juniper tree is a member of the cypress family, with all its associations of grief, betrayal, and death:*
>
> *Come away, come away, death,*
> *And in sad cypress let me be laid;*
> *Fly away, fly away, breath:*
> *I am slain by a fair cruel maid.*[2]

A story can state an existential dilemma briefly and pointedly, in a way which resonates with the listener's own inner conflicts, so they can imagine themselves healed and being whole.

Synopsis

A woman has a moment of joy at the birth of a son, then she dies. The boy gets a wicked stepmother, who knocks his block off, blames her own daughter, and cooks the boy in a stew for the father. The girl weeps and weeps and buries the boy's bones beneath the juniper tree, from which he emerges as a beautiful bird, singing of his fate. Then, singing a song, 'keewitt, keewitt, what a fine bird am I', the bird gathers a golden chain, a pair of fine shoes, and a millstone, imagining how they might be used. Returning home, he drops the gold chain round his father's neck, throws the fine shoes down for his sister, and drops the millstone on the terrified mother's head, knocking her block off. A happy ending for the boy, his sister, and his father.

The Story

Thousands of years ago there lived a good and beautiful woman, the wife of a rich man. They longed for a child. In the garden of their home stood a cypress, the juniper tree. One day in deep mid-winter the woman stood beneath the juniper tree peeling an apple, and her heart was sad. The knife cut her finger, and a few drops of blood fell on the snow. She gazed at it and said,

"I wish I had a child as white as snow and as red as blood." As she spoke these words, she felt moved within her and said to herself, "something will come of this."

She watched the seasons change, beneath the juniper tree, the coming of buds and fragrant blossoms and then the rich heavy fruit, as the life grew inside her. But when she saw the fruit hanging heavy on the tree, a change came over her. She grabbed the fruit greedily, cramming it into her mouth. She sickened. Her child was born, and the sight of him was a moment of exquisite joy, for he was as white as snow and as red as blood, as she had wished. Then she died.

The father wept a while and then took another wife, who gave birth to a daughter. The mother loved her daughter deeply, but her husband's son she hated. She pinched him. She slapped him. And when he reached out for her, she shooed him away and made him stand in shame in the kitchen corner.

One day the daughter came in and said,

"Mother, give me an apple." The mother opened a solid oak chest with a heavy iron lid where the apples were kept, took one out and gave it to her.

"And one for my brother too." At this the mother was vexed. She snatched the apple from her daughter's hand and put it back in the chest, saying,

"Then you can wait until your brother gets home."

Later the boy came in, and the mother said sweetly,

"My son, come and help yourself to a nice, juicy apple", and lifted the chest lid. The boy moved over to the chest warily. He looked from the smile on her lips to the juicy apples, to the look of hate in her eyes.

"Yes, I would like an apple, but how grisly you look." He leant into the chest to reach an apple, and, thwack, she brought down the lid and knocked his block off. His head rolled down among the apples.

"How can I shift the blame?" she thought. She sat him in a chair, balanced the head on the neck, tied it on with a white kerchief, and put an apple in his hand. Later the daughter came in and said,

"My brother is sitting holding an apple, but when I asked him for the apple he wouldn't reply."

"Ask him again", said the mother, "and if he still doesn't reply, slap him across the face." She went to her brother, asked for the apple, and when he didn't reply she slapped him across the face as her mother had told her. To her horror and dismay, the head bounced off and landed at her feet, the little eyes looking up at her.

Screaming and crying she rushed to her mother, who was stirring a pot over the kitchen fire,

"O mother, I've knocked his block off."

"What a dreadful and wicked thing to do," said the mother. "But it'll be our secret. We'll cook him up into a stew."

When the father came home, the mother said his son had gone to visit his mother's great uncle and he'd be gone for weeks. She served him the stew, while the daughter wept and wept.

"Mm," said the father, "I've never tasted such a delicious stew. Give me more, more, I'm going to eat it all up."

He gnawed the bones and threw them on the floor, and while the daughter wept and wept she gathered them all up in her silk kerchief. Still weeping bitterly she laid them at the foot of the juniper tree. Suddenly the roots of the tree shook, the branches parted and smoke, and steam and flames billowed out, and there came forth the most beautiful bird with a glorious lilting song. It flew high into the air and was gone. And the kerchief and the bones were gone.

Alighting one day on the roof of the goldsmith's house, the bird sang his glorious song:

My mother killed me. My father ate me.
My sister gathered my bones in a silken kerchief.
And laid them beneath the juniper tree.
Keewitt, keewitt. What a fine bird am I.

The goldsmith heard the song as he sat in his workshop making a golden chain and was entranced. Stepping over the threshold he called to the bird,

"What a wonderful singer, what a glorious song, give it to me again."

"Only if you will give me the golden chain you are holding."

"Willingly, willingly," said the goldsmith. The bird flew down and took the golden chain in his claw, and hovering before the goldsmith, he sang his song again.

The story relates how the fine bird flew to the shoemaker's house, and then to the mill, and received a pair of fine shoes in his other claw and a millstone around his neck for singing his glorious song to an admiring audience.

And so he lived his life as a bird, the golden chain in one claw, the fine shoes in the other, and the millstone around his neck, being admired by all as a fine bird with a glorious song. One day he returned to the house where he was born. His father and mother and sister were sitting at the table. He alighted on the juniper tree and began to sing his song.

"I suddenly feel so happy," said the father, "so light-hearted."

"I don't," said the mother with rising panic, "There is thunder in my ears, my eyes burn and flash like lightening." The sister just wept and wept.

My mother killed me.

"I'm so happy, the sun shines so bright, I feel I'm to be reunited with one I once loved."

"I don't. My teeth are chattering. There is fire in my veins." She tore open her bodice. The sister soaked the lap of her apron with her tears.

My father ate me.

"There's a beautiful bird out there, with a glorious song, and the air smells of cinnamon. I'm going out to see the bird close to."

"Don't go, don't go, the house is quaking and going up in flames." And the sister went on weeping.

My sister gathered my bones in a silken kerchief.

As the father stepped out, the bird dropped the gold chain around his neck, a perfect fit. Going inside, he said,

"See what a fine bird. He gave me this gold chain." But his wife had thrown herself on her back, with her legs in the air, screaming and panting in terror,

"If only I were a thousand feet underground and couldn't hear this song. I feel like the world is coming to an end."

And laid them beneath the juniper tree.

The sister leapt up,

"I shall go and see if the bird has something for me." The bird threw down the fine shoes. They landed near her feet. She stepped into them; they were a perfect fit. They danced her into the house with joy in her heart.

Keewitt, keewitt.

The woman dragged herself to her feet, her clothes ripped and her hair standing on end like tongues of flame. She staggered out of the house.

What a fine bird am I.

The bird dropped the millstone, and—thwack—it knocked her block off and squashed it flat. The ground shuddered and split open, and steam and smoke and flames shot out. Hearing the noise the father and sister rushed out. As the smoke cleared, where the millstone had fallen, beneath the juniper tree, there stood the boy, restored to his true likeness. Taking his sister and his father by the hand, they returned to the house to eat the meal and were all safe and very happy.

Source

This story is loosely based on the story *The Juniper Tree* included in *Grimms' Fairy Tales*.

Johnson, Stephen (1994), *Character Styles*. Jacob and Wilhelm Grimm, *Children's and Household Tales* (*Die drei Spinnerinnen, Kinder- und Hausmärchen*). The translation I have has the title *Grimm's Tales for Young and Old.*

Reflections

My Psychological Reflection

The Juniper Tree paints an accurate psychological picture of The Hated Child. The mother longs for a child. At his birth, the sight of him is a moment of exquisite joy. Then, she dies to him; the reality proves too much, the infant is too needy, too clingy, too messy, too demanding. She cannot give him the love he needs for his wellbeing. As she withdraws from his attentions, he learns that it's safer to keep his distance from her—and subsequently his detachment from other people in his life. He feels the absence of his mother's love and blames himself; his core belief is, 'I am flawed. There is something wrong with me.'

The Hated Child carries the covert belief, 'I am flawed. There is something wrong with me,' into adulthood, and compensates for it by creating the overt belief, 'I am a special person', to carry himself proudly into the world. This is the psychological split; just as in the story the boy compensates for being a hated child by transforming into a beautiful bird with a glorious lilting song,

"Keewitt, keewitt. What a fine bird am I."

At the other side of the split, the sister carries the split-off feelings of self-blame, grief, and loneliness, and throughout the story weeps and weeps, while the fine bird carries a millstone around his neck, his unconscious and unexpressed retaliatory rage. In traditional tales, it is unusual for the hero to kill his tormentor, but the hated child cannot be healed without uncovering his feelings of rage and grief and finding ways of expressing them in a safe, healing context.

The fine bird somehow knows that a second transformation must be undergone if he is to find safety. His life as a bird has been about gathering the inner resources needed to transform. When the crisis comes, in the story, the transformation is expressed in the mother's body with enormous intensity,

"I'm so afraid, my teeth are chattering, there is fire in my veins, there is roaring in my ears, my eyes burn and flash like lighting, the whole house is quaking and going up in flames, I feel as if the world is coming to an end."

It is a rebirth as orgasmic as birth itself.

Saint Corentin and the Golden Fish

Suitable to tell or read to older children

'Saint Corentin and the Golden Fish' is a deeply psychological story about the crisis of meaning, which people in mid-life are prone to endure. St John of the Cross (16th century) offers a profound description of the aridity of this crisis as a stripping of their faculties, the affections and feelings, spiritual and sensual, interior and exterior, leaving the understanding in darkness, the will dry, the memory empty, and the affections of the soul in the deepest affliction, bitterness and distress, withheld from the former sweetness it had in spiritual things.

The story is the healer; the story touches the Soul.

Synopsis

Friar Corentin lives in a clearing at the heart of a mighty Breton forest, spending his days praying and fasting. During his Lenten fast, desire for nourishment fills his aching body and soul. One morning, going to the spring pool to drink the cool water, he sees, swimming in the pool, there is a golden fish. He becomes tormented by the golden fish until one day he grabs the fish from the pool and pops it in the pot with onions and shallots and garlic. He eats the golden fish. Then he feels conscience-stricken, gathers up the bones, and throws them in the pool. Next morning, there to his delight, swimming in the pool, is the golden fish. For the rest of Lent, he observes his spiritual practice with a light heart and eats the fish with an easy conscience. Then, King Gradlon and his men, dogs, and horses, lost in the forest, crash into Corentin's clearing, demanding food with menaces. Friar Corentin responds to King Gradlon with quiet dignity, "Before this day is out, mighty king, thou shalt willingly bend the knee to the god of deer and hound," then feeds them all with onions, shallots, garlic, and golden fish, and Gradlon willingly bends the knee.

The Story

Friar Corentin lived in a small clearing at the heart of a mighty Breton forest. The trees bowed their branches low to form his hermitage, and the abundance of the forest provided for his needs. There was a spring in the clearing which never dried, trickling out into a hollow rock to form a clear and rippling pool.

He devoted himself to prayer and fasting, as his cloistered abbot had instructed him, in his search for the unseen god of wind and breath, allowing himself to enjoy the simple forest fare and the cool water of the spring pool.

One spring he began his long Lenten fast, as his cloistered abbot had instructed him, to subdue the flesh and to still its earthy desires. Each day was more tiresome than the last. The austere part of him struggled up the stony path of the spirit whilst desire for nourishment filled his aching body and soul.

On the seventh day of his fast, Friar Corentin rose just before dawn and went to the spring pool as usual to drink the cool water and to wash the sleep from his eyes. To the delight of his aching senses, he saw swimming in the pool a golden fish. The gold flooded out of the fish, filling the dawning forest with its light. And as the eyes of the fish rested upon Corentin, they rested him.

The fish delighted Corentin. He spent the day meditating upon it, measuring its length and breadth with his eyes, counting the very scales of its body, observing the subtle colours of its flesh and the rhythmic breathing of its gills, and celebrating its undulations through the rippling water. Delight.

As the days went by, the delighted part of him was captivated more and more by the golden fish, whilst the austere part became more and more demanding he return to the full, penitential rigour of his fast. As this struggle advanced, there grew in Corentin a desire for the golden fish. In his imagination he tickled its soft underparts in the way he had caught trout as a novice. He imagined grasping the fish and feeling it slithering in his fingers, its flesh oily and smooth and firm, the strange golden light radiating into his hands.

The austere part was strident, insisting the golden fish had been put into the spring pool by the god of fear and wrath for his temptation, to test him, to heighten his sense of mortification, if only he could overcome. In the depth of his struggle he prayed,

"Oh thou god of fire and tempest, keep me from temptation and preserve and protect the golden fish from my desires." Torment.

At noon on the 14th day, Corentin stood by the spring pool utterly, wearied by the struggle and strangely detached and still. As the eyes of the golden fish rested upon him, he reached into the water, lifted it out, and placed it in a pot which, in his detached way, he just happened to have warmed over the glowing embers of the fire he just happened to have made.

As the golden fish sizzled in the hot oil, he threw in onions and shallots and courgettes and sliced roots and rosemary and thyme and mushrooms and lots and lots of garlic. What savour filled his nostrils as the golden light irradiated the cooking pot? He remembered a bottle of fine Chateau Neuf his cloistered abbot had given him in a rare moment of generosity, opened it and began the finest breakfast he had ever known. The pot's bounty was unconfined and overflowing, and he ate and drank and enjoyed until he was perfectly satisfied.

Afterwards, he reflected on what he had done, the enormity of it. The golden fish had looked at him, and he had calmly and thoughtlessly grabbed it and ate it. What was worse, he had eaten it with great relish and enjoyment and had felt satisfaction and contentment. He was mortified. Ashamed. The austere part possessed him, calling him vile and weak and wicked and accursed for such a deed. And a tiny, tiny part of him said to itself,

"God, but it was good."

At the end of the day, forlorn and downtrodden by the austere part, Corentin slowly gathered up the head and tail and bones of the golden fish, walked to the spring pool and threw them in. Weary and beaten, he lay down and slept.

Friar Corentin rose just before dawn and went to the spring pool as usual to drink the cool water and to wash the sleep from his eyes. To his amazement and delight, there swimming in the pool was the golden fish. In that moment, he knew that the fish had been put there by the god of sowing and gathering, not for his temptation—or, not only for his temptation—but for his delectation and joy. Like the sheltering and abundant forest and the spring pool, the fish had been put there for his nourishment and for the comfort of his flesh.

He was a different person. Each day for the rest of the fast he observed his spiritual practice with a light heart and ate the fish with an easy conscience.

On the last day, there came a racket and tumult in the forest. With baying of hounds, whinny of horses, crashing of branches, howling of hunted deer, and coarse bellowing of men, there broke into Corentin's quiet clearing King Gradlon and 50 bold retainers, their horses steaming in the cool morning air. They had lost the quarry. She had escaped, sure-footed, into the dense undergrowth. King Gradlon was tired and hungry. He was angry and frustrated he had lost the prize of his manhood in the chase. Seeing Corentin, Gradlon turned his anger upon him,

"Thou, miserable little friar, give us all something to eat or I'll have thee flayed alive and carry thee home on a pole."

Gradlon's retainers listened with awe as Saint Corentin walked slowly towards the king, still astride his mount, looked him straight in the eye, and said,

"King Gradlon, thou art a mighty lord, but this is the land of one mightier than thou, the god of wood and stone. Here thou art his guest and mine. Welcome. I have olive oil and onions and shallots and courgettes and sliced roots and rosemary and thyme and mushrooms and lots and lots of garlic. I have the dregs of a fine Chateau Neuf. And I have one golden fish. With these I will serve thee a feast like thou hast never known. And before this day is out, thou, mighty king, shalt willingly bend the knee to the god of deer and hound."

The retainers sat silent on their steeds. No breath stirred. Save that the air fizzed and crackled between the two men as they confronted each other. Gradlon was a man without fear. He would wrestle with bears. As he absorbed Corentin's words, his hand moved to his bloodied sword. But he sensed a supernal strength in this slight saint, whose eyes rested upon him still, a strength like he had never met, that made him shift uneasily in his saddle and stay his hand. All the same,

"I shall make a bargain with thee," he said, with a great laugh to hide his unease, "A few weeds and one fish do not sound much of a feast to me. But, if thou canst feed me and all of my men until we are satisfied, I shall not flay thee alive and carry thee home on a pole."

The tension eased. King Gradlon and his men dismounted and stood around easily, making laughter. Corentin poured olive oil into his pot and set it to warm over the glowing embers. He gathered and prepared onions and shallots and courgettes and sliced roots and rosemary and thyme and mushrooms and lots and lots of garlic. He decanted the dregs of wine. Finally, he tenderly took the golden fish and put it in the hot oil with all the other ingredients. When the meal was ready, the king and all his retainers sat down to the greatest feast they had ever known, their palates enlivened by the most delicate flavours. The pot's bounty was as ever unconfined. The jug of wine was always overflowing. And they ate and drank and enjoyed until they were all perfectly satisfied.

In his amazement at such a feast, King Gradlon said how sorry he was to have struck such a bargain, asking what he might offer in recompense.

"There is one thing thou canst do," Corentin said, "Take the head and tail and bones of the golden fish and cast them into the spring pool."

As the king did as he was bid, before his eyes head and tail and bones came all together and the golden flesh reformed. As the eyes of the fish rested upon Gradlon, the king willingly bent his knee to the lively god, and all his retainers with him. And Corentin took the cool water of the spring pool and a little olive oil and anointed the brow of King Gradlon and all of his men in the name of the self-giving god.

Sources

Ashton, Agnes, 1975. *Saints and Changelings*, published by Blackie; Hillman, James, 1983. *Inter Views*, published by Spring Publications; St John of the Cross, 16th century. *The Dark Night of the Soul*. 1973 edition published by James Clarke.

The story of Saint Corentin and the Golden Fish comes from Breton mythology. The legend of *Saint Corentin*, the first bishop of Quimper, tells of a miraculous fish that regenerated itself after being eaten, which has parallels with earlier myths of gods who provided endless sustenance. https://lebarty.bongchong.com/breton-mythology/

Reflections

My Psychological Reflection

Crisis of meaning is all about soulmaking. It is both a cataclysmic life event and a process going on all the time. James Hillman (*Inter Views,* 1983) writes,

Soul makes the ego feel uncomfortable, uncertain, lost. Lostness is a sign of soul. You couldn't have soul or be a soul if you couldn't feel that you have lost it. The person in the strong ego doesn't feel he's lost anything. When whatever sustains ego cracks from inside, falls apart, so that we feel lost, weak, inferior, that is the sense of soul and the stuff from which soul is made.

Saint Corentin and the Golden Fish is the story of The Abandoned Child. Alone in a deep forest, Corentin has separated himself from the parental figure of the cloistered abbot. He has established his own ground. He can stand his ground. He has a solid sense of identity and manages his life with will and discrimination, allowing himself the simple fare of the forest and devoting himself to his chosen task. In his Journey of Soulmaking he has attained personal consciousness and will.

Yet, notwithstanding attaining much spiritual maturity, he betrays his psychological pathology, childhood abandonment and neediness, and his pre-personal issues in the way, as an ascetic monk, he denies his needs. Then, Corentin suffers a crisis of meaning.

In his extremity, Corentin reverts to the origin and deepest root of his psychological pathology, his childhood abandonment and neediness. He regresses to the ultimate fantasy of the needy child, the joy of both having his gingerbread cake—or golden fish—and eating it over and over again.

For Corentin, Soul is working on itself in the image of the golden fish, in the delight and the torment. The image, once he grasps it, is of a god who is at once self-renewing and self-giving, and in so being is the exemplar of self-realisation. With a secure sense of self, Corentin can greet pre-personal Gradlon with transpersonal Self-reflexive consciousness.

Notes

1 The 'enotes' website www.enotes.com/topics/maid-north/in-depth.
2 Shakespeare's words in *Twelfth Night*.

Bibliography

Afanas'ev, Aleksandr and Guterman, Norbert (Translator) (1945) *Russian Fairy Tales*, Pantheon Books. Copyright renewed by Random House (1973).

Ashton, Agnes (1975) *Saints and Changelings*, Blackie.

Grimm, Jacob and Wilhelm; Manheim, Ralph (Translator) (1978) *Children's and Household Tales (Die drei Spinnerinnen, Kinder- und Hausmärchen). Grimms' Tales for Young and Old*, Victor Gollancz.

Hillman, James (1983) *Inter Views*, Spring Publications.

Phelps, Ethel Johnston (1982) *The Maid of the North: Feminist Folk Tales from Around the World*, Holt Paperbacks.

Pinkola, Clarissa (1992) *Women Who Run with the Wolves*, Random House.

Schwartz-Salant, Nathan (1998) *The Mystery of Human Relationship: Alchemy and the Transformation of the Self*, Routledge.

St John of the Cross, C 16th *The Dark Night of the Soul* (1973 edition), James Clarke. Published 2003 by Dover Publications. First published January 1, 1584, with the original title, *La noche oscura del alma,* publisher unknown.

Original Stories Room

Original Stories are mainly Traveller's Tales that I wrote before I discovered psychosynthesis psychology, observation pieces that show some aptitude for qualities that subsequently serve me as a therapist.

Most of the stories in this book are my retelling of traditional stories. For each story, the overall plot is given, the words are mine. Since discovering traditional tales, I have only written two original stories, one of which is included in this collection; 'Once Upon A Time the Land Rejoiced As A Princess Was Born' blossomed out of an exercise in my psychosynthesis psychotherapy training.

Traveller's Tales

Before I discovered traditional stories, I wrote short observation pieces drawn from my life, brief encounters that I found moving, interesting, or full of meaning, or all of those things, including the following six stories. Several of my brief encounters have been on the London Underground, the least likely of places, including the next two tales.

Psychological Context for These Traveller's Tales

I wrote these tales before I discovered psychosynthesis psychology, so it's interesting for me, and hopefully for you also, to realise that these observation pieces show some aptitude for qualities that serve us as therapists: observation, empathy, imagination, humour, and even courage. Please, keep these qualities in mind as you read these Traveller's Tales.

For me, the quality of intuition came later.

DOI: 10.4324/9781003712329-12

The Man On the Up Escalator—A Christmas Story

This is the first story I ever wrote, many moons ago. I passed it round the office just before Christmas. The feedback I got from colleagues was, "Has this man finally lost touch with his senses?"

The Story

We see him on the Underground. He is riding the up escalators. He is in late middle age. We see his sober suit under a grey, well-cut gabardine coat. We see the firm line of his jaw. We see the short, well-groomed hair. Beside him we see his short, sober, grey-suited, well-groomed wife.

There are hundreds of us, riding the escalators, thousands. Our grey, intent faces are bunched in thought about nothing important, hurrying towards nowhere special. Riding the escalators with our dark, private thoughts of Christmas future. We would not have seen him, much less spared him a passing thought, as he rode the up escalators, sober and grey. Except for one thing. He wears a Father Christmas hat. Those of us on the up escalators stare up at him. Those of us on the down escalators crane around, jostling to gaze at his receding adornment. His slow progress up the escalators leaves a turbulent wake.

He wakes us fellow travellers from our preoccupation. He is a bow wave of curiosity and humour. He lifts the day. We feel gratitude and slow warmth. Here on the escalators, here in the press of a thousand bodies, is this single, scarlet flash of irrepressible humanity. We connect. We smile in response to the bobbing white of his greeting. He responds to our attention just with a gentle creasing of his eyes and a straight, quiet smile. It is a statement. Here is a man who does not take himself too seriously. Here is a man who can make himself conspicuous, the butt of popular humour, without loss of dignity or self-regard. The well-cut gabardine. The deliberate headgear. Here is his statement of freedom and independence.

Maybe he comes from lands afar, where customs differ, where people do not stand on the right when riding the up escalators. He stands on the left, beside his wife. There is a young man walking up the escalators. He is too preoccupied to be aware of the rising spirits around him. Briefly, he brushes against the man in the Father Christmas hat. There is a moment of confusion, the threat of altercation and ruin. Each of us is pierced by a sense of his fragility, the man in the Father Christmas hat. Each of us feels the puffed membrane of his self-regard and airy humour. It could so quickly burst open into mob derision and self-reproach. It could rob him of his casually borne independence. We draw and hold a collective breath. The moment passes. He is courteous. The thin line of his smile holds firm, unwavering. Amidst our alarms. We sigh. We know now; collectively, we feel the ground of his light assurance. His self-knowledge.

He passes up, off the escalators. He walks coolly out of our lives, arm in arm, as silently as he had come, in his Father Christmas hat. With us he leaves three gifts. His gift of impish humour to lift our spirits and lighten our Christmas darkness. His gift of awakening into a shared experience. His gift of knowledge, alive within us still.

The Girl With Green Hair

I sometimes have what I call Cameo Conversations, brief encounters with strangers. 'The Girl With Green Hair' is one of them.

The quotation, 'Do not seek death. Death will find you. But, seek the way that makes death a fulfilment,' is from the book 'Markings' by Dag Hammarskjøld, page 136. As Secretary General of the United Nations, in 1952 Dag Hammarskjøld commissioned a meditation room for people regardless of their faith. The meditation room remains in use. At the opening ceremony, Dag Hammarskjöld said: "We have within us a centre of stillness surrounded by silence. This house, dedicated to work and debate in the service of peace, should have one room dedicated to silence in the outward sense and stillness in the inner sense."

The Story

I am on a visit to London. I take the Underground, the Piccadilly Line train from Hounslow West to the city centre. The girl boards the Underground at Knightsbridge. She takes the seat next to mine. She has green hair. She crouches over a book. It is well thumbed and ragged edged.

I am preoccupied with my own thoughts and hardly notice her. Until she turns to me suddenly and asks,

"What's fumitory?" I ask her, what is the context? She says,

"It's in this book I'm reading for my A level exam. King Lear."

"Well," I say, "it's a herb. It means smoke of the ground."

But the last thing on her mind is etymology. She says,

"It has a terribly sad ending." There is a catch in her throat, "Everybody dies." The last syllable lengthens almost to a wail.

"Yes," I say—I am generalising in my mind—"everybody does die."

"But it's so sad." Again, almost a wail.

"In the story," I say, "Lear and Cordelia are reconciled before they die. They don't just die. They die reconciled. That's what's important about the story." But the last thing on her mind is literary criticism. She says slowly,

"Yes, but it's so sad."

I feel the sadness too. There is a pause. Then she says,

"Everything is dying around me. First my horse died. Then my cat died. Now my grandma has died."

She sits in her sadness for a few moments. I sit with her. We are quiet. Then,

"What do you think about death?" she asks.

I reply with words that have spoken to me,

"Do not seek death. Death will find you. But, seek the way that makes death a fulfilment."

"Yes!" she says, "Yes! That's it."

She nods her green head slowly. The train draws into Holborn. It's my stop.

At the Dove At Chiswick

> *Perhaps it's true; I really have finally lost touch with my senses, if this encounter is anything to go by.*

The Story

I am sitting nursing my pint of London Pride on the veranda of The Dove at Chiswick, vacantly gazing into the turgid, low-tide-turning Thames, when I hear a high-born, far-back voice pronounce,

"If those Liverpool supporters are so well behaved, why do they all carry knives?"

On an incautious impulse, I turn towards this Hurrah Henry, saying, in my pseudo-Scouse,

"I 'eard da'."

He takes the offensive. Leaning towards me, he flutes,

"I've been to Anfield, and those Liverpool supporters all carry knives. If they are so well behaved, why do they have knives?"

I lean forward towards him,

"De saw you comin'."

"Oh," he says, sinking back a little.

His friend, another Hurrah Henry, puts in a word of caution,

"I say old chap, watch out for this one, he has a glass *{long a}* in his hand."

At this point I seem to lose my presence of mind. Leaning further forward towards the Hurrah Henry and looking him directly in the face, I hear myself utter the words,

"D'yer wanna come outside er wha'?"

He sinks right back, hastily backing off,

"Frightfully sorry, old chap, fancy me making such a remark like that right next to the only scouser in the pub. Ha! Ha!"

"Da's a' right," I reply, leaning back myself, "We're famous for our sense of 'umour."

I slowly down my pint and quickly make myself scarce before I expose too much of my fake Scouse or a whole gang of Hurrah Henrys appear in the pub.

In Burlington Arcade

> *This story is about my encounter with a consummate professional.*

The Story

He greets me as I browse amongst the antique shops of Burlington Arcade.

"Oh, hello, how good to see you. Very handy actually."

"Oh, yes, good to see you too." Margery is always telling me I'm no good with faces, I ought to pay more attention.

"You're just up for the day are you, from ..."

"...from Brighton, yes." And it's good be on my own for a day. Much as I love you, Margery, I love you best when I'm on my own.

"You've left your wife at home for the day, have you?"

"Yes, Margery hates London, and can't stand trailing round galleries."

"No, Margery's more of a people person isn't she?"

"Yes, I suppose she is, coffee mornings and bridge in the afternoon."

"Oh, yes, and Margery's always so nice with my daughter, Alice, you'll have seen us loading her, in her wheelchair, into our car with its raised roof."

"Oh!"

"You know, I have a funny feeling you don't know who I am."

"Well ..." I am beginning to feel alarmed.

"I'm from Brighton, you must know me."

"Yes, of course, I ..."

"I live just down the road from you, in ..."

"...in Argyll Street? Oh, yes, well of course, that must be where I've seen you."

"Let me see now, you must be number ..."

"...yes, number 42."

"We're near the end, number 5. So, you remember me now." I frown, a little discomfited that he knows so much about me and I haven't the faintest idea who he is.

"I'm sorry, I wasn't sure. You know how it is when you recognise someone and you can't think where from, work, sports club ... I'm sorry I didn't recognise you straight off." God, what will Margery think of me?

"Oh, I understand. I'm terrible for faces. By the way, it is handy we met. I've broken down, and had to leave Alice, to find a phone box and ring the AA. I'm a bit worried. I'm not a member, you see, and they might not come out if I can't pay cash. You couldn't help me out could you?"

I hesitate, conflicted. A small part of me sees the con. A large part of me fears Margery's wrath when she hears I refused to help and turned him down.

He begins to back away, raising his palms,

"I'm sorry, I shouldn't have presumed. I'll sort something out, don't worry, don't worry."

I move towards him, I can't help myself,

"No, really..."

Well, I pay him ten pounds for the story. Or so I tell myself.

Dreaming of Place

> *Well, perhaps I have lost touch with my senses, but I have a fine, flowing connection with imagination.*

The Story

From the field brow, close to my home, the land slopes to the north and east down to sparse woodland and to the south and west to rolling pasture. In the southwest corner, Stroud Farm nestles in the hollow. It is an ancient farm site with an Elizabethan farmhouse and four other listed buildings. A local archaeologist tells me he once delved in the ground here for Anglo-Saxon history.

As I reach the field brow on my morning walk, I notice it stands in a circle of grass which is of a darker shade and a more lush texture than the surrounding field, like a fairy circle, I think. Then I see, or dream, an ancient tribe gathered at the field brow. Within the circle stands their queen, bearing a staff as tall and straight and strong as herself.

As I stand and watch, the queen hands a staff to me. It is as if they have been waiting for me. I stand in the circle, with my staff, at the field brow, facing the queen, with the tribe about us.

Now, each time I walk this way, I stand with my staff, facing the queen, with the tribe about us, sometimes drumming, or singing, or just talking and laughing. I feel privileged.

After a few weeks, one morning, as I reach the field brow, I see the tribe under attack and scattered all over the field. I can do nothing except stand with my staff and be witness to the slaughter.

The next day, the queen is being buried at the field brow by some of her tribe. Her face is serene. Her body is still tall and straight as she is gently laid in the ground. I stand solemnly with my staff.

Next time I walk this way, the queen's grave is covered, and beside it crouches a lone drummer playing a slow beat upon his drum. I stand in solemn sadness beside him with my staff.

Next time I walk this way, an ancient tribe is gathered at the field brow. Within the circle stands a chief, a thick-set man with a black beard and fierce countenance, bearing a staff. He demands the return of my staff, which I must proffer.

Next time I walk this way, and ever since, as I stand at the field brow, there is nothing to be seen but grass. Something is ended, is complete. Something is understood.

Dark Night of the Soul

> ***Warning!*** *Whilst this story is a faithful record of my encounter with five youths at the Castle public house, written straight after arriving home, it contains foul, prejudicial, and discriminatory language.*

Psychological Context

I invite you, a fellow therapist, to read the story despite my warning. Returning to this story after some years, I am struck by the divergence in the characters and feelings of these five young men, even though they dress alike, appear to have similar backgrounds and attitudes. Angus is a natural leader, confident, coarse, and cocky, yet with a certain courtesy and sense of pride. Bill is suspicious, maybe feeling threatened, a little menacing, and impulsive. Danny is hypersensitive to Charlie's shifting mood, calming him when he feels it necessary. Charlie, the oldest and least mature, boosting his poor self-worth with alcoholic aggression, with being Angus's lapdog, and with boasting of his full passport.

And what about me? Stealing their souls for print copy.

The Story

I walk to the Castle pub and order a pint of bitter. I take it into the garden and sit at a bench. It is a mid-summer evening with a warm breeze to lift my spirits. Music ambles across from the bar. Dire Straits. Brothers in Arms.

At a nearby table are Bill, Angus, Colin, Danny and Charlie. I don't learn their names till later. They wear old trainers, baggy shorts, tee shirts, and back-to-front baseball caps on their cropped heads. They are, though, very different in their uniformity, as I am to discover. They drink lager.

I settle down to my reading. *Dark Night of the Soul* by St John of the Cross. The work is slow. I sip my bitter. I carefully underline key passages.

Bill, Angus, Colin, Danny, and Charlie, their attention flits across the surface of the pub garden. They call across to people as someone catches their attention, "Like your shorts, mate, which jumble sale you get them in?"

At a glance, the subject of their curiosity turns away. Someone else,

"Come over here, love." She walks across and sits down. Angus speaks to her.

"~~Xxxx~~ off!", she stamps away, red faced.

Angus has the most to say, loudly. Sometimes he stands to call someone at a distant table. He catches sight of me with my book,

"What you reading?" I hold up the book.

"Dark Night of the Soul," his attention flicks away.

Bill moves towards the arched doorway of the pub to get in another round. He speaks to me as he passes my bench,

"He wants to know where you got those trainers." They are blue. New. I look up. Angus is looking at me.

I put down the book. I walk across to their table slowly. I am carrying my drink. My eyes are on Angus. His eyes are on me. I feel a thrill of uncertainty and anticipation.

"What do you want to know?" I sit down.

They all look at me. I wear an orange shirt. I like it, it was £10 in Top Man sale. They all look at me. Angus tells me their names. I look at them in turn. Each one solemnly stands and shakes my hand. I tell them my name. For a moment everything is still. Charlie speaks to me suddenly,

"I got my full birth certificate today." I look at Charlie. They stop looking at me and scour the garden. Except Charlie. He is very drunk.

I sip my bitter. A group of people enter the garden. One of them is a young woman. She has soft blond curls and tight black pants. Angus speaks to me,

"Has a ~~xxxxx~~ ever got in that ~~xxxx~~, do you think?"

{I leave you to fill in the blanks.

Mm! Well, I warned you about the language.}

What to say? Without breaking the spell.

"How am I supposed to know that?" They all laugh. They watch the young woman as she walks towards the doorway of the pub. I watch. Through the arch and out of their minds. They search out some new distraction.

I sip my bitter. I speak to Bill,

"Is this your local?"

"We drink here sometimes." He glances at me suspiciously and looks away.

"Where do you normally drink?" I persist.

"Don't know, lots of places." He stares across the garden. I feel menace. He wears a Union Jack tattoo on his arm.

Now Charlie is telling me his story. About the birth certificate,

"It's a full birth certificate. It has my mother's name on it and my father's name on it." He is maudlin. Sometimes he is aggressive,

"I could've just stayed with my little birth certificate. But I didn't. I got a full birth certificate and paid £15 for it." When he is maudlin they ignore him. When he is aggressive Danny speaks to calm him. Danny is hypersensitive to the tiniest shift in Charlie's mood.

I lean towards Charlie,

"Let me see your full birth certificate." He takes it from his trouser pocket. He unfolds it and hands it to me. His father is called Ronald and is a meat inspector. His mother is called Margerie, a shop assistant. Charlie is 35 years old.

I am still leaning forward. I look down at the birth certificate, open in my hands. I look up at Charlie,

"This seems very important to you."

"I paid £15 for one with my mother's name on it and my father's name. I didn't have to do that." Danny's radar pings.

"See this!" Danny takes hold of my wrist and places two fingers on my lower arm.

"This is white. He's one of us." He stares sideways into Charlie's face, a shoulder thrust forward. Charlie is maudlin again. Danny relaxes. He seems to ignore Charlie. I hand the birth certificate back to Charlie. He puts it on the table.

I sip my bitter. Charlie eyes my shirt, an orange shirt,

"Let's change shirts." He pulls off his tee shirt. It is green. "Ethnic!" is announced. "Save Mother Earth!" it insists. Why not! I unbutton my shirt and take it off. Bill grins at my body,

"I see you've been under the sun lamp," Angus says, "White man." Charlie dons my orange shirt. I put on his ethnic tee shirt. Danny watches carefully.

Time passes. I sip my bitter. Charlie talks about his birth certificate. Bill snaps, standing suddenly, knocking over his chair,

"I can't take any more of this!" He shakes my hand quickly. He shakes hands brusquely with Angus, Colin, Danny. Not with Charlie.

"~~Xxxx~~!" He walks away.

Charlie wanders off to the gents. I sip my bitter. He does not return. I sip more bitter. He still does not return.

"What about your shirt?" Angus's voice rises in concern.

"No big deal", I say, "it only cost a tenner."

"No, no, you must have it back." Something is at stake here, "I'll get it back for you."

Charlie has left his birth certificate on the table. Amidst the litter of empty glasses, crisp packets, and cigarette packs.

Once Upon A Time the Land Rejoiced As A Princess Was Born

Suitable for older children

> *This story began as a psychosynthesis psychotherapy training exercise to write a story beginning with the words, "Once upon a time the land rejoiced as a prince or princess was born." Surprisingly, I found myself choosing the 'princess' option. So, here is the story resulting from the exercise, 'Once Upon A Time the Land Rejoiced As A Princess Was Born.'*

Psychological Context

My plan for the story gradually emerged, with the princess being the narrator of a story about her little brother, my inner child, facing an adult world. Whilst the story is a fantasy, it does embody some of my inner child's challenges and his adversaries, dragons and vampires, with which he had to contend.

Synopsis

This is the story of a normal girl with a vivid imagination and how she feels like a princess, Princess Veronica. How she is born and how her land rejoices. This is her story. Oh, or Princess Veronica's story! As she would say, "Whatever!" It's about how she watches over her little brother Adam as he goes off on his Great Quest fighting dragons. How he is beguiled into entering the Circles of Enchantment to face his fiercest dragon foe. And is torn to pieces. Even then, she protects his spirit, and .... Whatever, just read it.

The Story

"Once upon a time the land rejoiced as a princess was born." This is how I like to begin my story. I think of myself as a princess. I really do. Not that I have a princessish name, Princess Veronica, but I can still feel like a princess, can't I? Well, I am as tall as a princess. I have short auburn hair, more of a pageboy than a princess, but anyway. I think I am as beautiful as a princess. I have a straight nose and grave grey eyes—I like that. I think I have quite high cheekbones, and my cheeks are flat underneath them, nearly hollow. I have a stern little mouth, anyway I think of it as stern, regal somehow.

Near to the palace where we live—it is in Paradise Street, the middle of three, and our Dad calls it a double-semi—there is a park, quite a large one, with an enchanted lake at the very centre. I love to walk alone in my park on windy days. In the autumn. It is my kingdom, my land.

I have a funny feeling inside me that goes up and down with the wind in the trees. I love to stand by the lake, perfectly still, and feel the wind going up and down in me, and feel the cold creeping up my legs and around my body so that it makes me shiver. I can catch the shiver and hold it there. It feels like forever. It makes my heart swell. I cannot describe it any more. It has no words.

Now that I think about it some more, Princess Veronica is not a bad name. After all, I am a fairy tale princess. Fairy tale princesses do not have normal names like Elizabeth or Mary, but they have interesting names. We are interesting people. Hum, Hum! We are very wise and old. We live for centuries. But we stay very beautiful, with our grave grey eyes that see so much.

Well, that is enough about me now. This story is about when I was born and how my land rejoiced. It must be a funny thing being born. I remember when my little brother Adam was born. I imagined him swimming about in our Mum's womb, now the dog paddle, now the butterfly crawl. I felt how lovely it was immersed in that warm pool. Not a thought. Not a care. Just that lovely womb feeling.

When he was born it was a different matter. He screamed. Did he scream! I felt how angry he was at being woken up. He still thrashed about with his arms and legs, but his warm pool had turned suddenly chilly. And I felt how frightened he was of the monstrous, lumpy shapes that now swam around him and bumped into him. The first thought he ever had was of his loss; the first conscious feeling was a stabbing pain. I understood somehow and watched over him.

His second conscious feeling was hunger. Wailing, overwhelming hunger, as the link with our Mum was cut. He could not tell the first loss from the second; they merged into one everlasting wail. Now he wails and works for his nourishment and plays hunt the nipple, for warmth and comfort and to keep himself alive. I know he does this, but not he. All he knows is what he must do to rid himself of those awful feelings, push them away. But they come back, they always come back, and he goes on driving them away.

With him it is just on with his armour and off to fight the foe. All those dragons that he sees! I watch and wait for him to come home like the patient princess that I am, but he does not see me. What boy does see his big sister?

Well, there are not many dragons in Paradise Street, so our Adam made them up in his head. They were real enough to the other kids, though. He made his dragons fly and breathe fire. The kids were terrified, but they always came back for more.

He had this idea in his head that dragons had great wealth and power that they had somehow stolen from him. And he must win it back. This is how his Great Quest came about. Our Mum said, "Don't scuff your new shoes," and our Dad said, "Don't be in late," and off he strode with spring in his step.

He quailed when he met his first dragon. It was an evil, scaly, Scottish creature, with bitter breath, by the name of McGowan. The fight was short, Adam's bright young blade against McGowan's caustic gall. The fight was inconclusive, but Adam and McGowan inflicted wounds on each other that were long in healing.

Years later Adam met McGowan again, diminished and spent, and showed him some kindness and curbed his sense of triumph. I felt close to him then.

There were many dragons. There was Victor the Mandible, with teeth as sharp as razors, who lorded over Adam for a while. And Hemlock Will, whose potions were deadlier than any blade. Adam had to join forces with Hemlock to defeat Victor, by giving him a sleeping draught and pulling his teeth. That was a great victory and very sweet to Adam. But I did not feel close to him then.

Adam was not alone in his Great Quest. There were always other ignorant folk eager to heed his tales of adventure and join battle alongside him. He always had his way with words.

As Adam fought battle after battle, he drew strength from his adversaries. His armour became tougher and stronger, his helm more emblazoned, and his sword more keen. Yet, within these defences he was ever that same little man that both quailed at McGowan and showed him kindness.

Adam's fiercest and final dragon foe was the Lessening Leech, who takes the form of an emaciated vulture, surrounded and protected by the Eighteen Circles of Enchantment. These give him beauty of form and raiment, the voice of seeming reason and wisdom, the protective arm of concern and comfort, and an air of innocent goodwill. Only those who fall victim to his spell and are drawn into the Circles of Enchantment discover the horror within and his voracious appetites; he who can draw blood from empty veins yet never add one ounce of flesh to his dread bones.

Adam and his companions befriended the Lessening Leech, ill prepared as they were for his beguilement. For years he travelled along their road or met with them along the way and made trade with them. Always courteous, he learnt their secret ways. Until one hard day they passed within the Circles of Enchantment, and he revealed his face, fell and foul.

With courage failed and bowels loosed they met him on the field of valour, with all his mighty host. Adam, soon divided from his friends, was pulled down and torn in pieces. They sucked him dry, boiled off his flesh for soup, ground up his bones for meal, and cast his vitals to the dogs.

But I kept his spirit from them, and he came at last, in the autumn, to the shores of the enchanted lake at the very centre of my park. He cast his worn blade into the lake. He removed his emblazoned helm. He threw his heavy armour to the ground. He let fall mail and mantle. He stood by the lake alone, at the end of his quest, his life drawn as thin as our postman's whistle.

Then he raised his head, drew a breath, smelt the air, and stood perfectly still. A strange feeling grew inside him that seemed to go up and down with the wind in the trees. He felt the cold creeping up his legs and around his body so that it made him shiver. He caught the shiver and held it. It felt like forever. It made his heart swell, and with all his new heart he made a wish beyond words.

I am a fair and fey princess. I granted the wish I had awaited for so long. I am the wish. In this consummation I am born, and all my land rejoices. So this is not, as Adam thought, the end of his journey. It is, as he now feels, just the beginning.

Try explaining that to our Mum and Dad.

Bibliography

Hammarskjöld, Dag, Auden, W. H. and Sjoberg, Leif (Translators), Carter, Jimmy (Preface) (1963) *Markings: Spiritual Poems and Meditations*, Vintage Books, 2006.

Storytelling With Children Room

These tales illustrate the creative power of storytelling with children, as well as illustrating my interactive style of storytelling with children

One of my greatest joys is storytelling with children. This Room is meant for those who might know the same joy: therapeutic storytellers, teachers, Girlguiding and Scouting leaders, and youth leaders. This Room is far from being an instruction book on how to tell stories to children. It is simply an illustration of my approach to storytelling with children. It's also a bundle of terrific stories to tell with children.

This is a selection of the tales I have oftentimes told to children. I only wrote the stories down for inclusion in this collection. I have sought, in the way I have written the stories, to convey something of how I tell them to children.

I have an interactive style of storytelling with children. I include the children—the listeners—as much as I can in the telling. Hence, I encourage them to interrupt, to make comments, and to add their bits to a story, often contributing creative and imaginative ideas. Hence storytelling <u>*with*</u> *children. Speaking and listening is an essential part of a school's curriculum, in which storytelling can make an active contribution.*

When I spend a day in an infant and primary school, I begin in Assembly, telling the tale 'The Three Spinners'. The whole school is actively engaged in the story, on its feet spinning flax, a lively and energetic start to the day. 'The Three Spinners' is lower down in this Room, then the stories follow the order I use as I tell my way through the school, with the stories for younger children first, then stories for older children.

DOI: 10.4324/9781003712329-13

The Creative Power of Storytelling With Children

As everything begins in the imagination,
healing begins in the imagination.

Psychological Context: The Story Is the Healer

The context for storytelling with children, as well as the sheer enjoyment for teller and listeners, is summed up in the maxim:

The story is the healer.

Telling tales has the power to inspire and to change lives, and at its heart the power is in the quality of relationship between teller and listeners. So, in the *Storytelling With Children* Room, 'healing' means helping to nourish children in their psycho-spiritual growth, expanding Spirit and deepening Soul.

Therapeutic storytellers, I invite you to read and tell the stories with this psychological context: the story is the healer; its power is in the quality of relationship between you and your listeners. When you are storytelling with children, nothing more is needed.

Here are some examples from my own experience of storytelling with children.

Karim Finds His Moment

I am telling tales to a reception class, and being unsure of the time, I ask,

"Do I have time for another story?"

Immediately, a young boy pipes up, let's call him Karim,

"I've got a Jungle Book story."

He tells the story beautifully, his voice expressive, and he uses his arms and hands for further expression. Afterwards, I say to the class teacher,

"That was wonderful, the way Karim told his story."

"Yes," replies the class teacher, "Karim, he never opens his mouth."

Through storytelling, Karim finds his voice.

The story is the healer
and serves as a container for each listener's Soul energy.

Evie Tells Her First Story

Marvellous storyteller Alan Woollard has a weekly booking to tell tales between courses at a Cornish farm restaurant. There we are in the barn, with a circle of straw bales to seat our audience. I am a visiting storyteller, Alan, and I take turns to tell.

Two-year-old Evie, sitting on a straw bale with her legs dangling, watches and listens intently. In the middle of one of my stories, Evie seizes her moment. She steps down from her straw bale and moves to the centre of the circle. There, she looks me in the eye and mimics my performance, waving her arms around and mouthing sounds—she doesn't have speech yet—and so we continue, she tells a bit, I tell a bit, until our tales are finished.

Evie tells her first story. Awesome. Beautiful.

The Wisdom of the Young

The right story holds up a mirror to the listener's existential experience, and it is this which brings healing and transformation.

I am telling the story of Pinonçita (below) to a Year 1 class, six-year-olds. I end the story with the words,

"And, when she got home, she was a normal sized child just like you or me." The little girl on the front row …

{There's always a little girl on the front row, it's like she follows me around, intent on making a monkey out of me, with a cutting comment or a sharp rebuke.}

… the little girl on the front row, with a deep frown, rebukes me,

"You're not a child, you're a grown up." The girl next to her comes to my rescue. She turns to her neighbour and says,

"Yes, but grownups have children inside them."

Oh! The wisdom of the young, it took me seven years of psychotherapy training to know this.

A story can state an existential dilemma briefly and pointedly, in a way which resonates with the listener's own inner conflicts, so they can imagine themselves healed and being whole.

Therapeutic Storywriting: April's Story

Therapeutic Storywriting allows children to write stories about the issues they face, without having to identify themselves.

Along with a Teaching Assistant, I work six sessions of therapeutic storywriting with four children in a senior school's special wing for children with educational and behavioural difficulties. We work quite well together, the children storyboarding, writing their stories, and talking about them. In the group is a 12-year-old girl, we'll call her April, who reveals through her stories the way her home is not child friendly.

Arriving for our final session, I learn that neither the Teaching Assistant nor our usual room is available, and I am left with the children in a room overlooked by other children from a five-a-side court. This is most unsettling for the group. They noisily act out, shouting, arguing, and name-calling. It's chaos for some time, with nobody listening to my attempts at pacifying the group.

Then, something happens. April stands forward in the midst of the hubbub and takes control. She speaks in a commanding voice,

"Right! Listen to what David is saying."

The children obey her, quieten down, and sit at the table, and we work together for the remainder of the session.

April had previously taken part without much enthusiasm. Now, at the end of the Therapeutic Storywriting programme, this young woman finds her spirit, her power, and her authority.

The Three Spinners

A tale to be told to children of all ages

> *I need to work on the plummy voices of the queen and crown prince, but the old crones' northern accent is second nature to this Lancashire lad.*

A story can state an existential dilemma briefly and pointedly,
in a way which resonates with the listener's own inner conflicts,
so they can imagine themselves healed and being whole.

Synopsis

Rose's mother wants her to spin flax. But she does not like spinning flax. When their argument is overheard by the queen, the mother tells the queen, "She won't stop spinning flax." The queen takes Rose to the palace, shows her three rooms of flax, and says, "If you spin all this flax you shall have the crown prince as your husband. You shall be a princess." Rose likes the prince, but she does not like spinning flax. This is Rose's dilemma.

The Story

Once upon a time, there was a girl who did not like spinning flax. Her name was Rose.

{I tell the listeners what flax is. Then I say, like this beautiful linen shirt I've got on.}

Her mother was always on at her to spin flax, but she always said,

"I do not like, spinning flax and I will not do it."

One day, they were having this big row, just as the queen was going past in her golden coach. When she heard the noise, she got out of her coach, went into the house, and said,

"What's going on here?" *{In a plummy, queenie voice.}*

The mother was too embarrassed to say, I'm shouting at my daughter because she won't spin flax, so she said,

"I'm shouting at my daughter because she won't stop spinning flax. She's spinning me out of house and home."

"Well," said the queen,"—*{still in her plummy, queenie voice}*—"she can come to the palace with me, I've got flax and to spare." And so it was.

{Was Rose pleased about this? NO-O!*}*

When they got to the palace, the queen showed Rose three rooms, all as big as this hall, full of flax. Then, she said to Rose,

"You're such an industrious girl,"—*{still in her plummy, queenie voice}*—"so when you have spun all the flax in these three rooms, you can have the crown prince to be your husband. You shall be a princess. I'll return later and see how you're getting on."

{Was Rose pleased about this? NO-O!}

Actually, Rose quite fancied the crown prince, but it would take her a thousand years to spin all that flax, and …

{… and what? SHE DID NOT LIKE SPINNING FLAX.*}*

Rose just sat down in the first room and wept, and wept, until the queen returned and said,

"Oh!, my dear, I suppose you're a little homesick, so I shall come back later."

Then, still weeping, Rose sat by the window, where she saw three old crones from some strange northern place coming down the road. They wore colourful, voluminous clothes and ridiculous hats. The first old crone had a foot the size of a great big bucket. The second old crone had a lower lip so large it came right down onto her chest. The third old crone had a thumb the size of a prize marrow. The three old crones stopped under the window where Rose was sitting weeping, and spoke to her,

"Ee, lass, what's up wi' thee?"

Rose told the three old crones all about not liking spinning flax, and about the three rooms waiting to be spun, and about marrying the crown prince if she did it, and how she fancied him. They said to Rose,

"Ee, lass, that's nowt to worry thee, we'll do t' spinning for thee. Mind, tha must invite us to thy wedding, tha must say we're thy cousins." So, in they came.

{At this point, I address the listeners: Right, we're all going to spin flax. Everybody, on your feet. Now, this half of the room, you're the first old crone, whose foot is the size of a? GREAT BIG BUCKET! You're going to do the treading. … I demonstrate … This half of the room, you're the second old crone, whose lower lip is? SO LARGE IT COMES RIGHT DOWN ONTO HER CHEST. You're going to do the licking. … I demonstrate … This half of the room, you're the third old crone, whose thumb is? THE SIZE OF A PRIZE MARROW. You're going to do the twisting. … I demonstrate … And every time you slap the table … I clap … another skein of the finest flax falls to the floor. Let's go. This half of the room, your doing the treading. … I tread … This half of the room, your doing the licking. … I lick … This half of the room, your doing the twisting. … I twist … And every time you slap the table, another skein of the finest flax falls to the floor. … I clap … In no time at all the flax in the room has been spun.}

The three old crones hid behind the heap of flax, tittering, as the queen returned,

"Oh! My dear,"—*{still in her plummy, queenie voice}*—"what an industrious girl you are. Now, let's move to the second room."

{So, the three old crones, that's you, start to spin flax again. Everyone spins as before.}

Then, Rose and the three old crones move on to the third room.

{The three old crones, that's you, start to spin flax again. Everyone spins as before. Then, you can sit down now and have a rest.}

The queen is overjoyed,

"Oh! My dear, this is wonderful, I shall call the banns for your marriage right away."

All the most resplendent people in the land attend the wedding breakfast, then who should arrive but the three old crones, in even more colourful, voluminous clothes and even more ridiculous hats. The queen greets them gracefully,

"You must be Princess Rose's cousins," and seats them at the top table with Princess Rose and the crown prince. The crown prince, who knows nothing of these strange cousins, is puzzled, saying to the first old crone,

"May I ask,"—*{in an even plummier voice than his mother}*—"why do you have a foot the size of a great big bucket?"

"Ee, lad," she replied, "I got it through treading, through treading."

"Ah! Mm! I see." Then, he said to the second old crone,

"May I ask, why do you have a lower lip so large it comes right down onto her chest, like that?"

"Ee, lad," she replied, "I got it through licking, through licking."

"Ah! Mm! I see." Then, he said to the third old crone—*{in an even plummier voice,}*

"May I ask, why do you have a thumb the size of a prize marrow?"

"Ee, lad," she replied, "I got it through twisting, through twisting."

Ah! Mm! I see." Then he turned to his bride, saying—*{in an even plummier voice,}*

"My dear, I want you to promise me something, that you'll never spin flax ever again, otherwise you'll finish up looking like those cousins of yours."

"Never spin flax? Oh! I don't know about that," replied Princess Rose, "you know how much I enjoy spinning flax."

"Please, my dear, as this is our wedding day, please, promise me that you'll never spin flax ever again, so you won't finish up looking like those cousins of yours."

"Well," Rose replied with a little frown, "just this once, I'll do as you ask."

So, this was how Princess Rose married the crown prince and never had to spin flax ever again.

{Was Rose pleased about this? YE-S! Give yourselves a clap for being such wonderful storytellers. We all clap. }

Source

This story is loosely based on the story *The Three Spinners* included in *Children's and Household Tales—Grimms' Fairy Tales* (*Die drei Spinnerinnen, Kinder- und Hausmärchen*) by Jacob and Wilhelm Grimm. The translation I have has the title *Grimm's Tales for Young and Old.*

Getting Rid of the Mice

A tale to be told to younger children

Let the story tell the story.
The story enables the listener to generate a new way of experiencing themselves, which at the outset is unknown.

Synopsis

The king has everything he could possibly want of creature comforts. Except for the creatures which cause him discomfort. He needs to know how to live with them.

The Story

The king's life had everything he could ever want: deep sofas, a comfortable king-size bed, a fine palace hung with sumptuous curtains, deep carpets, a great round table, and every kind of gorgeous food, especially cheese; the king loved cheese. There was just one thing that marred his life, the palace was overrun with mice. They lounged and scratched on the sofas, ran up the curtains, made nests in the carpets, and worst of all they scurried across the king's table and ate all the cheese. When the king got up in the morning, what did he find in his slippers? *{MICE!}*

The king called his wise men together and demanded,

"Do something about the mice." They mumbled and grumbled, then one a bit wiser than the rest had an answer.

{Who would they invite to rid the palace of mice? CATS! }

Well, that worked. But then the palace was overrun with cats. They lounged and scratched on the sofas, ran up the curtains, made nests in the carpets, and worst of all they scurried across the king's table and ate all the cheese. When the king got up in the morning, what did he find in his slippers? *{CATS!}*

The king called his wise men together and demanded,

"Do something about the cats." They mumbled and grumbled, then one a bit wiser than the rest had an answer.

{Who would they invite to rid the palace of cats? DOGS!*}*

Well that worked. But then the palace was overrun with dogs. They lounged and scratched on the sofas, ran up the curtains, made nests in the carpets, and worst of all they scurried across the king's table and ate all the cheese. When the king got up in the morning, what did he find in his slippers? *{DOGS!}*

{I invite the children to choose which animals they would invite in next, several times round, but save elephants to the last, almost.

Then, who would they invite to rid the palace of???? ELEPHANTS!*}*

They lounged and scratched on the sofas, ran up the curtains, made nests in the carpets, and worst of all they scurried across the king's table and ate all the cheese. When the king got up in the morning, what did he find in his slippers? *{ELEPHANTS!}*

The king called his wise men together and demanded,

"Do something about the elephants." They mumbled and grumbled, then one a bit wiser than the rest had an answer.

{Who would they invite to rid the palace of the elephants? MICE!*}*

Well, that worked, because as you know elephants are terrified of mice, and, in no time at all, all the elephants had been chased out of the palace.

After that, the king got to enjoy having mice lounging and scratching on his sofas, running up his curtains, making nests in his carpets, and sharing his delicious cheese. And when the king got up in the morning, what did he find in his slippers? *{MICE!}*

Source

This tale is based on the story *The King, the Mice and the Cheese* by Nancy & Eric Gurney (Random House, 1965).

The Hat Seller

Definitely a tale to be told to young children

Before I tell this tale, I recruit several listeners to come to the front, then I tell them, "You're a troop of monkeys," and practise them in making hooting monkey noises and scratching their armpits. I also have with me the bag of the old hat seller's beautiful (!!) hats.

The right story holds up a mirror to the hearer's existential experience, and it is this which brings healing and transformation.

Synopsis

A bevy of monkeys make a monkey out of a roving hat-hawker and his granddaughter. It's a generational thing.

The Story

The old hat seller spent his days wandering from village to village selling his beautiful hats ... *{like this lovely—actually monstrous—hat on my head.}* ... One day, in the heat of the midday sun, the old hat seller felt so weary he sat down under a mango tree and fell fast asleep. Above him, in the mango tree, was a troop of monkeys.

{That's you guys. The monkeys howl and scratch, and open the bag of hats and put them on.}

The howling and scratching awakens the old hat seller, who finds his bag of hats is empty. Looking up, he sees the troop of monkeys, all howling and scratching and wearing his beautiful hats. The old hat seller politely asked the troop of monkeys to return his hats.

{I ask the listeners, what do the monkeys do? THEY HOWL AND SCRATCH, STILL WEARING THE HATS.*}*

In a stern voice, the old hat seller again asked the troop of monkeys to return his hats.

{I ask the listeners, what do the monkeys do? THEY HOWL AND SCRATCH, STILL WEARING THE HATS.*}*

The old hat seller waves his fist at the troop of monkeys,

"Give me back my hats."

{I ask the listeners, what do the monkeys do? THEY HOWL AND SCRATCH, STILL WEARING THE HATS.*}*

Now, the old hat seller is so angry he grabs the beautiful hat from his own head and fiercely casts it to the ground. Then, all the monkeys do the same, taking off their hats and casting them to the ground. The old hat seller gathers his hats back into his bag and glumly heads for the next village.

A few years later, the old hat seller's granddaughter had taken over his hat-selling business. One day, in the heat of the midday sun, the old hat seller's granddaughter felt so weary she sat down under the very same mango tree and fell fast asleep. Above her, in the mango tree, was a troop of monkeys.

{I ask the listeners, what do the monkeys do? THEY HOWL AND SCRATCH, OPEN THE BAG OF HATS AND PUT THEM ON.*}*

The howling and scratching wakens up the old hat seller's granddaughter, who finds her bag of hats is empty. Looking up, she sees the troop of monkeys, all howling and scratching and wearing her beautiful hats. The old hat seller's granddaughter sternly demands the troop of monkeys to return her hats.

{I ask the listeners, what do the monkeys do? THEY HOWL AND SCRATCH, STILL WEARING THE HATS.*}*

Then, the old hat seller's granddaughter remembers the funny story her grandfather liked to tell about how he got the better of a troop of monkeys. She takes off her own beautiful hat from her head and fiercely casts it to the ground. The alpha female monkey slowly climbs down from the mango tree, gives the old hat seller's granddaughter a sly grin, and says,

"So, you think you're the only one with a grandfather who tells tales."

Source

I don't remember where I heard this wonderful tale, but the Story Museum (www.storymuseum.org.uk/) tells us: This ancient Indian story comes from a collection of animal parables called *The Panchatantra*, which was first written down in about 300 BCE, interconnecting tales about jackals and elephants, tigers and crows.

The Golden Bowl

A tale to be told to younger children

This is a delightful tale to tell, with the children joining in the repeated lines:
A present for me, a beautiful golden bowl; give this bowl to the one you love the best; along the corridor, down the stairs, through the great hall…
I use a brass singing bowl as my beautiful golden bowl and let the children hold it and turn it over.

The story is the healer; the story touches the Soul.

Synopsis

The presence of a beautiful golden bowl touches the soul of the palace.

The Story

The King was grumpy, grrr—*{let's have some grumpy faces}*—Because the King was grumpy the Queen was grumpy, grrr. Because the Queen was grumpy the gatekeeper was grumpy, grrr. Because the gatekeeper was grumpy the kitchen maid was grumpy, grrr. Even the King's dog was grumpy, grrr woof. Everyone in the land was grumpy, grrr. One day, a messenger arrived at the gatehouse and said to the gatekeeper,

"I have a present for the King."

The gatekeeper took the present and went along the corridor, down the stairs, through the great Hall, across the courtyard, up the stairs, and along the corridor to the King's room and knocked on the door—*{knock, knock}*. The King opened the door and with delight he said,

"A present for me, a beautiful golden bowl." He admired the golden bowl, then turned it over and read the words underneath,

"Give this bowl to the one you love the best."

"Well," said the King, "that will be my dog." And he filled the bowl with water and placed it in front of his dog, who went woof, woof. Then the King stopped and thought,

"Ah, I suppose the one I love the best would be the Queen." So, the King went along the corridor, down the stairs, through the great hall, across the courtyard, up the stairs, along the corridor to the Queen's room, and knocked on the door—*{knock, knock}*. The Queen opened the door and with delight she said,

"A present for me, a beautiful golden bowl." She admired the golden bowl, then turned it over and read the words underneath,

"Give this bowl to the one you love the best."

"Ah," said the Queen, "well, that would be the King, but I can't give it to him because he has just given it to me. I know, I shall give the golden bowl to the gatekeeper. So, the Queen went along the corridor, down the stairs, through the great hall, across the courtyard, up the stairs, along the corridor to the gatekeeper's room, and knocked on the door—*{knock, knock}*. The gatekeeper opened the door and with delight he said,

"A present for me, a beautiful golden bowl." He admired the golden bowl, then turned it over and read the words underneath,

"Give this bowl to the one you love the best."

"Ah," said the gatekeeper, "I know who I love the best, and that's the kitchen maid." So, the gatekeeper went along the corridor, down the stairs, through the great hall, across the courtyard, up the stairs, along the corridor to the kitchen maid's room, and knocked on the door—*{knock, knock}*. The kitchen maid opened the door and with delight she said,

"A present for me, a beautiful golden bowl." She admired the golden bowl, then turned it over and read the words underneath,

"Give this bowl to the one you love the best."

"Well," said the kitchen maid, "I know who I love the best and that's the King." So, the kitchen maid went along the corridor, down the stairs, through the great hall, across the courtyard, up the stairs, and along the corridor to the King's room, but the door was open and the King was not there, so the kitchen maid left the golden ball on the table for the King to find when he returned. Later, the King saw the golden ball and said to his dog,

"Well, what a wonderful journey this beautiful golden bowl must have made around the Palace, so now I can give it to the one it was meant for all along, and he filled the bowl with water and placed it in front of his dog, woof, woof."

Now the King was happy—*{let's have some awful grimaces}*—and because the King was happy the Queen was happy—*{awful grimaces}*—and because the Queen was happy the gatekeeper was happy—*{awful grimaces}*—and because the gatekeeper was happy the kitchen maid was happy—*{awful grimaces}*—even the King's dog was happy, woof, woof, everyone in the Kingdom was happy—*{awful grimaces}*—and has been happy ever after.

Source

I don't remember where I heard this story. It may have been the delightful storyteller and musician Pippa Reid.

Pinonçita, The Very Little Girl

A tale to be told to children young and old

> *By the way, Pinonçita's breakfast with just one oat came from a 7-year-old listener, and I've used it ever since.*

Let the story tell the story.
The story enables the listener to generate a new way of experiencing themselves, which at the outset is unknown.

Synopsis

Pinonçita is a very little girl. When her mother goes out, she warns her daughter not to venture in the field behind the house, but Pinonçita seeks adventure and out she goes. That's how the very little girl begins her adventure into the unknown.

The Story

Once upon a time, there was a little girl, a very little girl, a very-very little girl, a very-very-very little girl. Her name was Pinonçita. Her mother had sewn a tiny-tiny-tiny dress for her and had forgotten to remove her tiny-tiny-tiny needle from its shoulder. Pinonçita had a tiny-tiny-tiny porridge bowl for her breakfast, just one oat with a tiny-tiny-tiny drop of milk.

One day, Pinonçita's mother said to her,

"I'm going to the shops, and while I'm out, you mustn't go into the field behind the house, it's too dangerous for a very-very-very little girl." But, when her mother had gone, what did Pinonçita do?

{Yes! She went out into the field behind the house.}

She wanted an adventure. It was wonderful in the field. The grass was so tall it was like walking through a forest. The bees around the bright flowers were frighteningly fantastic. She saw a worm worming by, like a huge dragon.

Then it began to rain, its drops as big as she was; she was going to be drenched. So, she took shelter under a mushroom, where she could watch the rain falling with such pleasure.

Then, pools of rainwater began to form around the mushroom. Pinonçita was a bit scared she might fall into a huge pool and drown. So, she put her arms around the mushroom's trunk to keep safe and enjoy life in the forest.

Then, Pinonçita saw a woman with a basket collecting something from the ground.

{Guess what it was. MUSHROOMS.*}*

The woman got closer and closer, then she picked Pinonçita's mushroom and put it in her basket, with Pinonçita still clinging to it. The woman took the basket home to her cottage. She built a fire under her great cauldron, poured in rainwater, along with onions and garlic and herbs, and the basketful of mushrooms and…?

{What was she cooking? MUSHROOM SOUP.*}*

Pinonçita was dog-paddling around in the great cauldron, as the mushroom soup got hotter and hotter. The woman took a great ladle, stirred it around in the mushroom soup, and brought out an overflowing ladleful of mushroom soup, with Pinonçita paddling around in it. As the ladle rose toward the woman's mouth, Pinonçita looked right up into her huge, hairy, horrible nostrils, then into her mouth with its terrible yellow tongue and broken, blackened teeth. The woman poured the ladleful onto her yellow tongue, and the slimy soup with Pinonçita floating in it slid down towards her gullet. Just before she slid down the woman's throat, Pinonçita saved herself by grabbing the little waggly bit at the back of her mouth.

{Do you have a little waggly bit at the back of your mouth?}

Grabbing the little waggly bit made the woman cough—*cough*—flinging Pinonçita out of her mouth, through the open window, and she fell onto the grass outside.

Pinonçita was rolling around on the grass, trying to clean off the mushroom soup. Nearby, there was a donkey gobbling grass. When the donkey came close to Pinonçita, he gobbled up Pinonçita as well. Pinonçita found herself sliding down towards the donkey's gullet, but the donkey didn't have a little waggly bit to grab hold of, so she slid right down into the donkey's tummy. It wasn't nice down there, landing in a heap of half-digested grass. She wondered to herself, how am I going to get out of this?

{The listening children are not slow to help Pinonçita get out of the donkey's tummy, but their answers are not repeatable here.}

Pinonçita remembered that donkeys' tummies are ticklish, so she tickled the donkey's tummy from inside, and the beast began to laugh, hee-haw, hee-haw.

{I encourage the listening children to make donkey laughing hee-haw, hee-haw noises.}

The donkey laughed so much he brought up his breakfast, splosh, onto the grass, with Pinonçita in the middle of it, the mushroom soup now coated in rotting grass.

Pinonçita was rolling around on the grass, trying to clean off the mushroom soup and rotting grass. A passing mummy blackbird thought she saw a particularly plump juicy worm to feed to her chicks. She flew down and picked up Pinonçita in her beak. Pinonçita was crying out,

"I'm not a fat, juicy worm, I'm a little girl," so the mummy blackbird took Pinonçita back to her nest and her chicks. She looked at Pinonçita,

"You don't look very happy, have you had very much food today?"

"No," replied Pinonçita, "only a bit of mushroom soup and some rotting grass."

"Well," said the kindly mummy blackbird, "I shall go and get you something to eat. How about some nice fat juicy worms? Please, look after my chicks while I'm gone."

Pinonçita was telling the chicks all about her adventures when she espied a sly snake sneaking silently down the branch towards the nest. She thought of a picture she'd seen of a snake having eaten a sheep, with a sheep-shaped bulge along its back, and imagined a row of chick-shaped bulges. What could she do to defend the chicks?

{I ask the listening children, what can she do? Maybe someone will remember the needle in the shoulder of her dress.}

She remembered the needle her mother had left in the shoulder of her dress. She flourished the needle, threatening the snake not to come any closer. With a disappointed sneer the snake sidled off, just as the mummy blackbird returned and saw how bravely Pinonçita had saved her chicks.

"Oh, my dear," she cried, "what can I do to repay you?"

"Take me home," pleaded the little girl.

"Climb on my back, and I will carry you home in a couple of ticks," she told her.

The kindly mummy blackbird carried Pinonçita to a short distance from her home, telling her what she must do,

"Find a little bone, and roll it forward in front of you, and with each roll you will be a little bit bigger."

So, Pinonçita found a bone that was almost as big as she was, and when she heaved it forward she became a little bit bigger. As she rolled the bone forward, each time she rolled it forward it got easier as she got a little bit bigger, and when she got home she was a normal-sized child just like you or me.

Source

Pinonçita, The Very Little Girl is based on a traditional story from Chile. In the traditional tale, after the mother has been given a pinon fruit to bring her luck, she gives birth to a very little boy, *Pinonçito*. In the present version, it's a very little girl, and the story starts some time after her birth.

The Crystal Ball

A tale to be told, or read, to children young and old

I have told this story so many times, and as I now write it down I realise it is a story that cries out to be told to young listeners. So, please, practise this story, develop the characters, in your use of voice and movements, and in the way you dialogue with the listeners so that, as you tell the tale in your unique way, the listeners become part of the oral storytelling tradition.

As everything begins in the imagination,
healing begins in the imagination.

Synopsis

A young man takes flight from his witch of a mother, his imagination fuelled by the most beautiful woman in all the world.

The Story

Once upon a time, there lived a powerful sorceress who had three sons. She loved her sons dearly, but she feared that they would steal her book of spells and become more powerful than she, so she turned her eldest son into a sardine, and she turned her middle son into a pigeon.

When he saw it was likely he'd be turned into something, maybe a flea, her youngest son, who was The Little Big Fellow, went off on his travels.

{I use a funny voice when I say, The Little Big Fellow.}

In his travels far and wide, he heard about The Most Beautiful Woman in All the World, who was held captive by an Evil And Wicked Sorcerer, in the Palace of the Golden Sun, at the top of the Crystal Mountain, beside the Silver Sea.

The Little Big Fellow searched for seven years to discover The Most Beautiful Woman in All the World, and at last he found the Crystal Mountain. He walked a few steps up the Crystal Mountain, then slid down to the bottom again, time and time again. Then, he noticed lots of brave Knights and their horses scattered about the foot of the Crystal Mountain, moaning and groaning in agony. Each one had galloped towards the Crystal Mountain hoping to reach the summit and to discover The Most Beautiful Woman In All the World, but after a few strides they lost momentum and slithered to the bottom in a whimpering heap.

The Little Big Fellow said to himself, Hm! I shall need to think about this overnight and went off into a nearby forest. Early the next morning, in the forest, he met three trolls: two men trolls and one gigantic woman troll.

{I ask the listeners, do you know the troll song? Yes? No? Well, let's sing the troll song anyway. I show everyone the lumbering, rolling actions.

I'm a troll fol-de-rol
I'm a troll fol-de-rol
I'm a troll fol-de-rol
I'll eat you for my supper.

Well, this has nothing at all to do with the story, but I enjoyed it, hope you did.}

The gigantic woman troll seemed to be in charge. She looked pleased to see the Little Big Fellow, and going up to him she said …

{I speak with a funny, cockneyish, deep troll voice.}

"You look like an intelligent sort of chap. We have this problem, see, and you can help us decide what to do, see. We have this magic cap, see, and when we put it on and say we want to go someplace, then we go someplace, see. But we don't know whose turn it is next, and we're arguing about it, see. That's our problem, see, so will you help us?"

Well, the Little Big Fellow was not at all interested in their problem, but he said,

"Oh, well, just give me the cap, then I'll walk to that tree over there, and when I say ready, steady, go, you run to me and the one who gets there first gets the next go with the cap."

The gigantic woman troll's face shone with pleasure—as far as a troll face can shine with pleasure—"What a good idea," she said.

The Little Big Fellow began to walk towards the tree, but all the time he was wondering how to get to the top of the Crystal Mountain while absentmindedly putting the cap on his head.

{I ask the listeners, what do you think happens next? I talk with the listeners. The tale goes on. Yes, he found himself at the top of the Crystal Mountain in the Palace of the Golden Sun.}

And, he had solved the trolls' problem as well—they didn't need to argue any more.

He searched every room in the palace looking for The Most Beautiful Woman In All the World. He searched 999 rooms without finding her. Then, in the 1000th room, there she was. He said to her,

"You're supposed to be The Most Beautiful Woman In All the World, but you look awful, your hair is a tangled mess, your face is covered in warts, you are dressed in rags, and your teeth are sitting in a jam jar by the side of the bed." She was quite put out and replied,

"What do you expect me to look like at 6 o'clock in the morning? Anyway," she went on, "The Evil And Wicked Sorcerer has put me under a spell to make me look like this. If you want to see how I really am, you have to see me through that mirror." The Little Big Fellow looked in the mirror and saw The Most Beautiful Woman In All the World in all her glory. Her skin was the colour of honey. She had rich, deep golden hair. She wore a beautiful blue gown adorned with all the stars in the heavens. Her teeth were like fine alabaster, sitting in a jam jar by the bed.

{What, you expect miracles?}

Then she said, "If you want to rescue me from The Evil And Wicked Sorcerer, this is what you have to do. Go to the bottom of the Crystal Mountain. There you'll find a bull with massive horns. So, kill a bull. Out of the bull will fly a firebird with a red-hot egg inside it. The yolk of the egg is the Crystal Ball. Make the firebird lay the egg, but don't let the egg reach the ground otherwise it will burst into flames, the Crystal Ball will melt, and all will be lost. Hold up the Crystal Ball in front of The Evil And Wicked Sorcerer and he will lose his power over me."

{I got all that? Well, have you got all that? You'd better tell me, to be sure.}

The Little Big Fellow went sliding down the Crystal Mountain—the quick way, wheeee!—At the bottom of the mountain he saw the bull. He killed the bull.

{Well, I could spend two hours telling you how he killed the bull. Do you want me to do that? You do? Well I can't, I've got a bus to catch. The tale continues. }

The firebird emerged from the bull and flew up, and up, and away. The Little Big Fellow couldn't catch it. He thought all was lost. Then, he saw a great eagle flying down from high above.

{Guess what! What's going to happen? Talk with the listeners.}

The middle brother, who'd been turned into a … *{ask the listeners}* … pigeon, had grown up to be a great and mighty eagle. The eagle harried the firebird, making it lay the egg. The egg fell down, down, down towards the sand beside the Silver Sea. Once again, The Little Big Fellow thought all was lost.

{Guess what! What's going to happen? Talk with the listeners.}

The eldest brother, who had been turned into a … *{ask the listeners}* … sardine, had grown up into a great and mighty whale, rising up from the Silver Sea. With one flick of its mighty tail, a great tidal wave extinguished the red-hot egg, an inch before it burst onto the ground. The egg cracked open. Revealed inside was… *{ask the listeners … THE CRYSTAL BALL.}*

The Little Big Fellow went back up the Crystal Mountain. *{How did he do that?}* He stood in front of The Evil And Wicked Sorcerer, and holding up the Crystal Ball, he said,

"With this Crystal Ball I take away your power over The Most Beautiful Woman In All The World."

"Oh, rats!" said The Evil And Wicked Sorcerer.

"Now," said The Little Big Fellow, "is your chance to be a Kind And Helpful Wicked Sorcerer by marrying me to The Most Beautiful Woman In All the World, if she's willing." Which she was.

And so it was, The Most Beautiful Woman In All the World and The Little Big Fellow and The Kind And Helpful Wicked Sorcerer lived happily ever after, in the Palace of the Golden Sun, at the top of the Crystal Mountain, beside the Silver Sea.

Source

This tale is loosely based on the story *The Crystal Ball*, one of Grimms' fairy tales. *Children's and Household Tales—Grimms' Fairy Tales* (*Die drei Spinnerinnen, Kinder- und Hausmärchen*) by Jacob and Wilhelm Grimm. The translation I have has the title *Grimm's Tales for Young and Old.*

The Well of the World's End

A tale to be told or read to children young and old

> *This is one of the best tales to tell interactively with a class or group of children. Because there's plenty of repetition for the listeners to join in and best of all there's a song for everyone to join in singing. You'll have to make up your own tune.*
>
> *The Well of the World's End is a Scottish tale, so when I tell it I put on a fake Scottish accent for the words spoken, which is actually quite good, but it doesn't have to be; it's probably best as an obvious fake. You can have fun with the little frog's croaky voice.*
>
> *Actually, adults enjoy this tale too. I once told it at a house-warming party, singing the words in the song 'my honey my heart'. Afterwards, one of the guests suggested I use the Gaelic 'mo hinny mo croí' instead, which I've done ever since.*

The story is the healer
and serves as a container for each hearer's Soul energy.

Synopsis

Orphan Moira is sent for water from the Well of the World's End by her unkind stepmother. For a water container, she is given a sieve and told not to come home without the sieve being full of water. At the Well of the World's End, Moira meets a little frog, who tells her how to fill the sieve with water, and in return she promises to do everything he asks of her all day and all night long. The little frog proves to be a bit of a pest, but it's a fairy story, so it works out well in the end.

The Story

Moira was an orphan, and, as happens in fairy tales, she had an unkind stepmother, who gave her a hard time. One day, the stepmother decided to get rid of Moira altogether, saying to her,

"Tak' this sieve to the Well of the World's End, and dinna bring it back till it's full o' water."

{I ask the listeners what a sieve is, some don't know.}

Moira happily trotted off to look for the Well of the World's End, asking everyone she met,

"Please, where can I find the Well of the World's End?"

But they all shook their heads. Moira became ever more hungry and weary. Then, she met a wise old woman, bent double with age, and asked her,

"Please, where can I find the Well of the World's End?" The old wise woman knew the answer,

"Ay, lassie, go over the hill and down the dale and there ye'll find the Well of the World's End." Moira went over the hill and down the dale and there she found the Well of the World's End, set about with Spring flowers and with crystal clear water. Moira happily plunged the sieve into the water and brought it out, and …

{What happened? ALL THE WATER POURED OUT.*}*

… then she tried again, and …

{What happened? ALL THE WATER POURED OUT.*}*

Moira unhappily sat on the edge of the well and wept and wondered what to do, for she couldn't go home till the sieve was full of water. Then, she heard a croaky voice,

"I'll tell ye how to fill the sieve wi' water, if you promise to do everything I ask of you all day and all night long." Moira saw a little frog sitting beside her. Well, she thought, it shouldn't be too hard to do what a little frog asks of me, so she agreed, and the little frog began to sing,

"Pack it wi' moss and smear it wi' clay,
And then ye can carry the water away."

So, Moira packed the sieve with moss and smeared it over with clay, then plunged the sieve into the well and brought it out …

{What happened? THE SIEVE WAS FILLED WITH WATER.*}*

Moira was so delighted she forgot all about the little frog but rushed away home, without hearing the little frog singing behind her,

"Remember the promise ye promised to me,
At the World's End Well this morning."

The stepmother was surprised and displeased when Moira happily burst in carrying the sieve full of water. She just took the sieve into the back kitchen, and nothing more was said.

Later, Moira and her stepmother were having their dinner when there was a tap, low down on the door. The stepmother looked up and told Moira to see who it was. When Moira answered the door …

{Guess who it was on the doorstep. THE LITTLE FROG.*}*

The little frog began to sing,

"Tak' me in, mo hinny mo croí,
Tak' me in, mi' darlin',
Remember the promise ye promised to me,
At the World's End Well this morning."

{In case you didn't know, mo hinny mo croí means my honey my heart. So, all together, in a croaky voice, TAK' ME IN, MO HINNY MO CROÍ...*}*

"Tak' me in, mo hinny mo croí,
Tak' me in, mi' darlin',
Remember the promise ye promised to me,
At the World's End Well this morning."

Moira shut the door, leaving the little frog on the step, and went back to the table.

"Who was that?" asked the stepmother, and Moira had to tell all about the little frog and the promise she had made. The stepmother said,

"A promise is a promise, a girl must keep her promises. Let him in."

So, Moira let the little frog in, and it hopped—hop, hop, hop—up to Moira's chair and began to sing,

{All together, in a croaky voice ...}

"Pick me up, mo hinny mo croí,
Pick me up, mi' darlin',
Remember the promise ye promised to me,
At the World's End Well this morning."

"Ugh! Ugh! A slimy frog on my nice clean apron. Ugh!" But the stepmother said,

{What? "A PROMISE IS A PROMISE, A GIRL MUST KEEP HER PROMISES. PICK HIM UP."*}*

So, Moira picked up the little frog, and the little frog began to sing,

{All together, in a croaky voice...}

"Gimme my dinner, mo hinny mo croí,
Gimme my dinner, mi' darlin',
Remember the promise ye promised to me,
At the World's End Well this morning."

"Ugh! Ugh! A slimy frog on my nice clean plate. Ugh!" But the stepmother said,

{What? "A PROMISE IS A PROMISE, A GIRL MUST KEEP HER PROMISES. GIVE HIM HIS DINNER."*}*

So, Moira picked up the little frog and put it on the corner of her plate, the little frog began to eat Moira's dinner, slurping up the food with his long tongue, slurp, slurp. The little frog was now a big little frog, and the big little frog began to sing,

{All together, in a croaky voice...}

"Tak' me to bed, mo hinny mo croí,
Tak' me to bed, mi' darlin',
Remember the promise ye promised to me,
At the World's End Well this morning."

"Ugh! Ugh! A slimy frog on my nice clean bedclothes. Ugh!" But the stepmother said,

{What? "A PROMISE IS A PROMISE, A GIRL MUST KEEP HER PROMISES. TAK' HIM TO BED."*}*

So, Moira picked up the big little frog, carried him up the winding stairs to her bedroom, and put the frog in the bed on one side, then climbed in on the other side, as far from him as possible.

Early the next morning, Moira heard singing,

{All together, in a croaky voice...}

"Chop off ma head, mo hinny mo croí,
Chop off ma head, mi' darlin',

Remember the promise ye promised to me,
At the World's End Well this morning."

"Ugh! Ugh! Green frog's blood all over my nice clean bedroom. Ugh!" So, the frog sang again,

{All together, in a croaky voice...}

"Chop off ma head, mo hinny mo croí,
Chop off ma head, mi' darlin',
Remember the promise ye promised to me,
At the World's End Well this morning."

Then, Moira heard her stepmother's voice in her head,

{What? "A PROMISE IS A PROMISE, A GIRL MUST KEEP HER PROMISES. CHOP OFF HIS HEAD."*}*

So, Moira went down the winding stairs to the woodshed, bringing back the biggest axe she could carry. The frog squatted on the floor, sticking his neck out for the axe as far as it could go. Moira lifted the axe high in the air, shut her eyes very tight, and brought down the axe with a thud. With her eyes still firmly shut, she heard singing,

{This time I sing in a rich baritone voice—if you can believe that.}

"Come to my arms, mo hinny mo croí,
Come to my arms, mi' darlin',
Remember the promise ye promised to me,
At the World's End Well this morning."

Moira opened her eyes, and there before her was…

{What? A HANDSOME PRINCE. *This time, without any reluctance whatsoever, she leaped into his arms.}*

The frog, of course, had been under a spell. And so, Moira and the handsome prince lived happily ever after,

{Where? THE WELL OF THE WORLD'S END. *Where else?*
Give yourselves a clap for being such wonderful storytellers. We all clap.}

Source

This is the Scottish version of *The Frog Prince.* It can be found in English Fairy Tales (ed. Steel, Flora Annie, First Edition 1918).

The Greatest Gift

A tale to be told, or read, to older children

We sin against the imagination when we ask a story for its meaning.

Synopsis

A magic telescope, a magic carpet, and a magic lemon are gifts brought for brothers Tammy, Timmy, and Tommy by their much-travelled uncle. These gifts enable the brothers to travel to a far country to save the life of a princess, in return for a bag of gold and the hand of the princess in marriage. They can share the gold, but with three brothers and only one hand, whom shall she marry?

The Story

Magic! Magic! Magic! Once upon a time, there were three brothers, Tammy, Timmy, and the youngest, Tommy. Their rotund Uncle Tummy travelled the world, and every time he arrived home he had a magical present for Tammy or Timmy or Tommy.

When Uncle Tummy got home from Shanghai, he brought a present for Tammy.

"Thank you uncle," said Tammy … *{without enthusiasm}* … "just what I've always wanted, a metal tube with a bit of glass at each end."

"Ah, replied Uncle Tummy, "it's not just a metal tube with a bit of glass at each end. It's a telescope, and not just a telescope, it's a magic telescope. When you look through the telescope, you can see things happening thousands of miles away."

When Uncle Tummy got home from Istanbul, he brought a present for Timmy.

"Thank you uncle," said Timmy … *{without enthusiasm}* … "just what I've always wanted, a scruffy old carpet."

"Ah, replied Uncle Tummy, "it's not just a scruffy old carpet, it's a magic carpet. When you sit on the magic carpet and say you want to go some place, you go some place."

When Uncle Tummy got home from Timbuctoo, he brought a present for Tommy.

"Thank you uncle," said Tommy … *{without enthusiasm}* … "just what I've always wanted, a lemon."

"Ah, replied Uncle Tummy, "it's not just a lemon, it's a magic lemon. When you feed slices of this lemon to someone who's sick and fit to die it makes them better."

One day, Tammy is looking through his magic telescope, and behold, thousands of miles away he sees a king holding up a bag of gold,

"My daughter Princess Petal has the squirrel flu and is fit to die. I'll give this bag of gold and my daughter's hand in marriage to anyone who can make her better."

{This is just a story, but kings really did marry off their daughters, once upon a time. }

"Pity we've no way of getting there," said Tammy to Timmy and Tommy, "or we could have gone to help."

"But we can," replied Timmy excitedly, "we can go on my magic carpet." So, they all climbed aboard the magic carpet and said where they wanted to go.

{I pause here, ask, "Has anyone been on a magic carpet?" Sometimes, someone says they have, so we talk about it. Then I go on, "The thing about magic carpets, they don't have a petrol tank, so they use themselves for fuel." I hold up a very, very small carpet. "This used to be the size of this hall, but I've used it so much, it now can't lift a flee." Then I continue the story. }

The magic carpet cruised above the ground at a breathtaking pace, to the immense excitement of Tammy, Timmy, and Tommy, till a great oak loomed up right in their path,

"AAH!" they yelled. Slipping right and leaning left, the magic carpet expertly powered around the great oak like a powerful motorbike, and the next, and the next, it was exhilarating. Ahead, a tall mountain, and whoosh,

"AAH-AAH!!" they yelled. Flying almost vertically, the magic carpet folded around them to keep them onboard. A moment's respite as they turned the summit, then the rapidest rollercoaster ride down the other side,

"AAH-AAH-AAH!!" they yelled, leaving their stomachs far behind.

Now on the flat, the magic carpet scorched ahead at ever-increasing speed. It was then that Tammy, Timmy, and Tommy discovered what else the magic carpet lacked.

{What do you think it is? Talk about it. Then…}

A windscreen! There was no protection from bugs, flies, wasps, crows, or even the occasional cow, plastering them from head to foot. When they arrived at the king's palace they looked—and smelt—like something the cat brought in.

They stood together before the king. He looked them up and down, twitched his nostrils, raised his nose, and spoke,

"Shove off, we don't want smelly urchins like you in our nice, clean kingdom." Tommy bravely stepped forward, looked the king in the eye, and replied,

"Your kingliness, we have heard that your daughter Princess Petal has the squirrel flu and is fit to die, and we are here to make her better."

The king lowered his nose a trifle and ushered Tammy, Timmy, and Tommy into Princess Petal's bedchamber, where she lay moaning and covered in sticking plasters, looking pale and wan, with her hair all limp. She looked down her nose at them and screeched,

"What are you doing in my sick room? Don't you know I have the squirrel flu and am fit to die? I don't want smelly urchins like you in my nice, clean bedchamber…." She went on screeching in this fashion. Each time she paused for breath, Tommy popped a slice of his magic lemon into her mouth. She screeched, and he popped lemon. She screeched, and he popped lemon. Slowly, colour returned to her cheeks, her hair recovered its lustre, and the magic lemon had made her better. She went on and on shrieking.

The king was overjoyed,

"You have made my daughter Princess Petal better. Thank you, thank you. Here is the bag of gold to share between you." Then he bethought himself, "Oh, I promised Princess Petal in marriage to whoever made her better, but which of the three should it be, Tammy, Timmy, or Tommy?"

"Not me!" declared Tammy, Timmy, and Tommy all together.

> *{Well, I think we should let the audience decide. If it wasn't for Tammy's magic telescope they would never have known about Princess Petal's squirrel flu. If it hadn't been for Timmy's magic carpet they would never have got there. If it hadn't been for Tommy's magic lemon Princess Petal would never have got better. So, which should she marry, they're all keen to aren't they? Aren't they? So let's put it to the vote.*
>
> *So that's what we do. It's usually a shambles. Some want her to marry Uncle Tummy. Whatever, in the end I let the audience know whom she should marry.}*

Tammy still has his magic telescope. Timmy still has his magic carpet. But Tommy no longer has his magic lemon; he used it to make Princess Petal better. So his is the greatest gift.

Source

This tale is loosely based on the story *The Three Princes and the Princess Nouronnihar* from *The Arabian Nights.*

The Naming of Cuchullin

A tale to be told or read to older children, especially adolescents

Before the ending of 'the troubles' in Northern Ireland, I visited a fellow member of my Psychosynthesis Psychotherapy training cohort in the Falls Road, a staunchly republican area of Belfast. Perhaps this was not such a wise visit for an Englishman of Protestant heritage. My colleague showed me round the Belfast sites, including a painting on an end-of-terrace wall depicting the Irish hero Cuchullin, surrounded by paramilitaries bearing Armalite rifles. She let me take in the painting for a few moments, then she said quietly, "It's a Protestant wall."

The right story holds up a mirror to the hearer's existential experience, and it is this which brings healing and transformation.

Synopsis

King Conor, on his way to an ale feast in honour of his blacksmith Culann, is impressed by the hurling skills of a boy, Setanta, and invites him to attend the feast, then forgets. Arriving at Culann's castle, Setanta finds the gate locked and the castle guarded by a fierce watchdog. A fight to the death ensues between Setanta and Culann's ferocious cur, with an unexpected, life-transforming outcome.

The Story

King Conor was strolling along, anticipating a sumptuous ale feast with his friend and blacksmith Culann. As a master craftsman and the maker of the king's swords, Culann's renown was second only to the King himself. King Conor paused in his stroll to watch his Boy-Corps playing a game of hurling. The teams seemed to the king to be unevenly matched, with 12 boys on one side and only one boy on the other. Yet Setanta, as was the boy's name, being swift and nimble, scored many goals against his opponents, with nary a one between his own goalposts. King Conor's chest so swelled with pride to have such verve and talent in his Boy-Corps, he promptly invited the boy to come to the feast when the game was over. Then, he continued his stroll. And forgot!

After the game, Setanta made his way to Culann's castle, wielding his hurley and batting his ball against the castle wall. Meanwhile, King Conor, Culann, and the warriors of the king's Red Guard were ranked around the banqueting hall, ready for the feast. Culann spoke to the King,

"If all are assembled, sire, I will unleash my watchdog to guard the boundaries of my estate and lock the gates of the castle." With a casual wave of his hand the King thoughtlessly gave his consent.

Culann's watchdog is a sleek and mighty hound, a strong and savage cur, equal to a hundred other dogs. Approaching the castle gate, Setanta comes face to face with Culann's cur, all slavering jaws and thunderous growl, its bark sharp as lightning. Hearing the hubbub, King Conor, Culann, and the warriors of the Red Guard rush to the ramparts.

Taking a stance, weight on his front foot, hurley raised, Setanta stands his ground. Culann's cur, observing Setanta's firm grasp of his hurley, moves forward with caution, then lunges wide-jawed for Setanta's shoulder. With well-balanced precision, Setanta swings sideways whilst delivering a sharp, swift blow to the exposed shoulder of Culann's cur. Setanta and Culann's cur warily circle each other, shrewdly testing and observing each other with surprise forays, inflicting wounds without gaining advantage.

Gradually, there grows in Setanta and in Culann's cur a deep respect for each other's fortitude and courage. Yet, Culann's cur is bound to guard the boundaries of his master's estate at whatever cost and can do no other, and Setanta is bound to defend the Boy-Corps, including himself, at whatever cost and can do no other. Both are bound to continue the conflict, regardless of their growing respect for one another.

With Setanta holding up his hurley defensively in both hands, Culann's cur lowers his great head before making a sudden lunge for Setanta's body, intent on throwing him off balance before striking open-jawed for his face, but Setanta rolls backwards onto his back foot, creating room for a savage blow to the side of his adversary's head. For a few moments Setanta and Culann's cur gaze into one another's eyes, until the hound's eyes empty, his legs give way, and he sinks to the ground.

Setanta falls to his knees in pain and grief, placing his hand on the hound's head. A grief-stricken Culann walks from the castle and, looking down gently, places his hand on Setanta's shoulder. Above them, on the ramparts, the Red Guard are shouting and cheering with delight at such a victory.

Looking up at Culann, with tears in his eyes, Setanta speaks to him,

"I shall be the cur of Culann. I shall guard the boundaries of his estate."

And thus has he been named ever since, the cur of Culann, Cuchullin. Above them, on the ramparts, the Red Guard are shouting, 'Cuchullin, Cuchullin, Cuchullin.'

Sources

From *Irish Sagas and Folk-Tales* by Eileen O'Faolain, Oxford University Press, 1954.

My Psychological Reflection

The Naming of Cuchullin is a coming-of-age story, as well as a tale about repentance and atonement.

Your Psychological Reflection

I invite you to reflect on the moment you recognised your coming of age or remember making a clear and maybe difficult choice, and the emotions arising in you; on a moment when you may have felt the need for repentance and how you may have sought to atone, or been unable to atone, and the emotions arising in you.

Bibliography

Grimm, Jacob and Wilhelm; Manheim, Ralph (Translator) (1978) *Children's and Household Tales (Die drei Spinnerinnen, Kinder- und Hausmärchen). Grimms' Tales for Young and Old*, Victor Gollancz.

Gurney, Nancy and Eric (1965) *The King, the Mice and the Cheese*, Random House.

O'Faolain, Eileen (1954) *Irish Sagas and Folk-Tales*, Oxford University Press.

Steel, Flora Annie (1918) *English Fairy Tales*, published 2022 by Generic. (publisher of 1918 edition unknown)

Ending: The Meaning of Life

Lauren, the editor of this book, invited me in her wisdom to write an ending piece. She gave me the opportunity to set this book in a broad context, including some passages from earlier in the book.

Around 1,200 years ago my Danish Viking ancestors settled in Lancashire, where they worked the common land for many centuries until, by an Enclosure Act of the English Parliament, they were expelled. The men wanted to fight, but in order to survive, the wise women led the families away from the land into the town of Preston and into the dark satanic mills.

My maternal grandparents worked in a cotton mill, living in a mill worker's cottage with a front room, a kitchen, and a narrow kinked staircase up to two bedrooms. There was no bathroom, only a zinc bath in the yard, along with a wash house and an outside lavatory. As in every mill worker's cottage, there was the one precious item brought from the land, their milking stool.

My grandparents still lived there when I was a young child. My grandad was an especial influence on me, sitting with me and telling stories from his life. In the 1920s and 1930s he was the secretary of the Preston and District Cricket League. Every Sunday morning, many men crammed into their front room to talk about the 50 cricket matches that had taken place the previous day, while Granddad moved among them listening to their stories. In the afternoon, he wrote reports of all 50 cricket matches and took them to the offices of the Lancashire Daily Post for publication the following day. His motto was, do it now. It is with his commitment and determination that I have been able to write this book, with its essential cycle of submission, astute feedback, referral, and invitation to resubmit from publisher Susannah. When Granddad retired, feeling at a loose end, he did what he had sworn never to do; he crossed the threshold of the moribund Brackenbury Road Old Men's Brotherhood. And took charge.

I'm in my fifth year in secondary school. I make a list of the subjects I stand a chance of qualifying in, where my effort will be applied, which doesn't include geography. At the end of the autumn term, my geography teacher Mr Warburton says to me in open class, "England, you're going to fail this examination if you're not careful." Just this! It awakens a new confidence in me. I pass in geography. At year end, my head teacher (aka Bachus) writes in red ink on my annual report, "It

DOI: 10.4324/9781003712329-14

is a waste of time England going into the 6th Form." But, with the sustained confidence inspired in me by Mr Warburton, I do so anyway. Mr Warburton's gift is part of the social heritage, which with my genetic and familial heritage—Grandad saw and heard me and I've always seen him as my saviour—has served to shape the person I am.

My view of my life used to be just birth and everything in between until death. I now see this singular view as being too self-centred. My view of my life now, from a transpersonal perspective, is as part of a continuum, as a unique, separate, and independent life within the whole flow of human existence and beyond. Within this flow, as well as my genetic and familial heritage, I inherit from many who have been a significant influence, like Mr Warburton, and I am here to provide a legacy to those who follow after. The words of Dag Hammarskjöld (1963, p. 136) ring true for me, "Do not seek death. Death will find you. But seek the road which makes death a fulfilment." For me, this is the meaning of life.

From a transpersonal perspective—life as part of a continuum—death can be seen as a *relinquishing of life*. Over recent decades, there has been a shift of attitude from black-suited grief to the colourful raiment of celebration, as we look back, as we recall the life of the departed. At the same time, *relinquishing of life* suggests a looking forward, as we ask ourselves, "What inheritance do we receive from the departed, what insights and qualities do we take forward in fulfilment of our own lives." So it flows.

Bibliography

Hammarskjöld, Dag, Auden, W. H. and Sjoberg, Leif (Translators), Carter, Jimmy (Preface) (1963) *Markings: Spiritual Poems and Meditations*, Vintage Books, 2006.

Sting in the Tale

You may have noticed, I promised you 50 tales and I have only given you 49.
Well, the 50th tale is for you to write!

DOI: 10.4324/9781003712329-15

Index

Note: Page numbers in *italics* refers to figures and books.

The Abbess' Coif 11, 72–6
Advanced Research Projects Agency Network (ARPANET) 113
Afanas'ev, Aleksandr 161, 168
Always Look on the Bright Side of Life 144
The Arabian Nights 233
Armstrong, Annette 83
Ashton, Agnes 189
The Aspects of Being Human 21
Ātmabodha (Shankaracharya) 143, 144
At the Dove At Chiswick 14, 196
authentic mirror 32, 33, 35

Bawdy Tales 4–6, 9–12, 49–90; *The Abbess' Coif* 11, 72–6; *The Crane's Leg* 11, 50–3; *Cynethryth Queen of the Mercians* 11, 64–6; Defiant Saxon Queens 63; *Demeter and Persephone* 11, 59–62; intention 3; *The Laydys of the Towne* 11, 54–8; *Pearl of Wisdom* 12, 86–90; psychological/egalitarian reflection 49; *Queen Emma's Ordeal By Fire* 11, 67–71; *Sir Gawain and the Green Knight* 11–12, 77–85
Beastly Tales 4–6, 9, 10, 12, 47, 92–127, 129–30; *The Dun Cow of Parlick* 12, 108–13; *The Great Hairy Toe* 12, 114–7; intention 3; *King Gaarge and the Dragon* 12, 98–102; *Lady Sybil and the Milk White Doe* 12, 118–21; *Mr Fox* 12, 103–7; *The Unsworth Dragon* 12, 93–7, *96*; 'Witches' 129–30; *The Witches of Windsor* 12, 122–7
Bee, Mantis, and Flower 38, 39
Benjamin, Walter 63
Bettelheim, Bruno 3, 40
Bluebell Blessing (Holliday) 27
Boccaccio, Giovanni 52, 74
body 23, 26, 36, 62, 71
Bonn, Scott 106
Buddha 143, 144

Callimachus 140
carer of soul 33, 35
Character Styles (Johnson) 41, 184
Children's and Household Tales (Grimm and Grimm) 184, 213, 226
Clarke, James 189
Constructing the Sexual Crucible (Schnarch) 84
The Crane's Leg 11, 50–3
Creation Myth of the San People 7
The Creative Power of Storytelling With Children 208–10
crisis of meaning 189, 190
The Crystal Ball 15–6, 223–6
Cynethryth Queen of the Mercians 11, 64–6

Dark Night of the Soul 15, 200–2
The Dark Night of the Soul (Clarke) 189
The Dark River 29
The Decameron (Boccaccio) 52, 74
Defiant Saxon Queens 63
Demeter and Persephone 11, 59–62
differentiation 31–4, 62
Dream Dilemma 12, 133
Dreaming of Place 15, 199
The Dun Cow of Parlick 12, 108–13
The Dynamic Portrayal of Soul 9, 18–9, 23, *24*, 36; body 23, 36; feelings 23, 36; mind 23, 36; spirit 23, 36

Earthtales, Storytelling in Times of Change (Gersie) 140, 152
ego development 32
energy for life 24–5
English Fairy Tales (Jacobs) 105
Erysichthon and the Grove of Demeter (Callimachus) 140

False Foxes (Westwood) 105
The Feeling In Her Bones 14, 43, 177–80
feelings 23, 26, 36, 62, 71
fellow traveller 35
feminine energy 26–7
The Firebird and Princess Vasilisa (Afanas'ev) 168
The Four Elements 19, 20, *20*, 36
The Frog Prince (Scottish version) 230

gatekeeper 35
gender diversity 5
Gersie, Alida 140, 152
Getting Rid of the Mice 15, 214–5
The Gifts of Being Human 21–30
The Girl Who Loved to Dance 8–9, 11
The Girl With Green Hair 14, 194–5
The Golden Bowl 15, 218–9
The Greatest Gift 16, 231–3
The Great Hairy Toe 12, 114–7
grieving process 62
Grimm, Jacob 184, 213, 226
Grimm, Wilhelm 184, 213, 226
Grimms' Fairy Tales 184, 213, 226
Gurney, Eric 215
Gurney, Nancy 215
Guterman, Norbert 161, 168

Hammarskjöld, Dag 35, 238
Hardy, Thomas 4, 44
The Hat Seller 15, 216 7
healing power 7–9
Helping Children Cope with Loss and Change (Seyderhelm) 6
Hillman, James 25, 26, 38, 39, 189
Holliday, Susan 27
Holmwood, Clive 6
The Horse of Power 14, 163–9

In Burlington Arcade 15, 197–8
integration 31–4, 62
intercourse 26
Inter Views (Hillman) 189
Irish Sagas and Folk-Tales (O'Faolain) 235
Iris—Rainbow Goddess 13, 141–2

Jacksties, Sharon 6
Jacobs, Joseph 105
The Japanese Fairy Book (Osaki) 149
Jennings, Sue 6
Johnson, Stephen 41, 184
The Journey of Soulmaking 9, 18, *30*, 30–5; differentiation 31–4; ego development 32; integration 31–4; model in mirrors 31–5; personal consciousness and will 32–3; personal self 32–3; pre-personal consciousness and will 32; psychotherapy with soul 35; self-realisation 33–5; survival self 32; transpersonal consciousness and will 33–5; tri-focal vision 35
The Juniper Tree 14, 181–5

The King and the Oak 13, 139–40
King Gaarge and the Dragon 12, 98–102
The King, the Mice and the Cheese (Gurney and Gurney) 215

Lady Sybil and the Milk White Doe 12, 118–21
The Laydys of the Towne 11, 54–8
List of Creation Myths, Wikipedia 7
Lowes, Joanne *96*

The Maid of the North: Feminist Folk Tales from Around the World (Phelps) 174
Malone, Edmond 105
The Man On the Up Escalator—A Christmas Story 14, 192–3
masculine energy 25–7
The Master and His Emissary (McGilchrist) 57
McGilchrist, Ian 57
Medicine Wheel 18–9, 23, 24, 31
The Merry Wives of Windsor (Shakespeare) 127
mind 23, 26, 36, 62, 71
Monty Python's Life of Brian 144
Mr Fox 12, 103–7
Much Ado About Nothing (Shakespeare) 105
The Music and Story Experience with Pippa Reid 137
My Life on the Road (Steinem) 4
My Lord Bag of Rice 13, 146–50

The Naming of Cuchullin 16, 234–6
A New Gestalt: A New Way of Experiencing Ourselves 39

O'Faolain, Eileen 235
Once Upon A Time the Land Rejoiced As a Princess Was Born 15, 203–6
Original Stories 10, 14–5, 191–206; *In Burlington Arcade* 15, 197–8; *Dark Night of the Soul* 15, 200–2; *At the Dove At Chiswick* 14, 196; *Dreaming of Place* 15, 199; *The Girl With Green Hair* 14, 194–5; *The Man On the Up Escalator—A Christmas Story* 14, 192–3; *Once Upon A Time the Land Rejoiced As A Princess Was Born* 15, 203–6; Traveller's Tales 191
Osaki, Yei Theodora 149
An Owned Child 42–3

The Panchatantra 217
pathology 25, 26
Pearl of Wisdom 12, 86–90
Perry, Grayson 4
personal consciousness and will 32–3
personal self 32–3
Phelps, Ethel Johnston 174
Pinkola Estés, Clarissa 179, 180
Pinonçita, The Very Little Girl 15, 220–2
Pope, Alexander 4
A Portrait of Soul 1, 4, 9, 18–37, 71; The Aspects of Being Human 21; The Dynamic Portrayal of Soul 18–9, 23, *24*; The Four Elements 20; The Gifts of Being Human 21–30; The Journey of Soulmaking 30–5; Sexuality: Consciousness and Will 35–6; Songs of Being Human 36–7; What I Mean by 'Soul' 18
pre-personal consciousness and will 32
Principles of Transpersonal Psychology (Gilot) 30
psychotherapy with soul 35
"Purveyors of Deep Insight" 3–4

Queen Emma's Ordeal By Fire 11, 67–71

Reality and Imagination 39–40
receptiveness and intimacy 26–7
The Resonance of a Story 42–3
Routledge International Handbook of Therapeutic Stories and Storytelling (Holmwood, Jennings and Jacksties) 6
Rushworth, Terry *109*
Russian Fairy Tales (Afanas'ev) 161, 168

Saint Corentin and the Golden Fish 14, 186–90
Saints and Changelings (Ashton) 189
Salt Doll (Sri Ramakrishna) 145
Schlosser, S.E. 116
Schnarch, David 84
Schwartz-Salant, Nathan 89
self-realisation 33–5
self-reflection 32–3
self-reflexive consciousness 132, 145
Sexual Aspect 23
sexuality 23–7; consciousness and will 35–6; definition of 24; energy for life 24–5; evolution of 24–5; feminine energy 26–7; masculine energy 25–7; metaphor for 25
Seyderhelm, Amanda 6
Shamanic Wheels and Keys (SwiftDeer Reagan) 19, 22, 23
Shankaracharya 143, 144
The Sin Against the Imagination 39
Sir Gawain and the Green Knight 11–12, 77–85
Sir Gawain and the Loathly Lady 14, 170–5
Skeleton Woman (Pinkola Estés) 179, 180
Songs of Being Human 36–7
soul: definition of 18; inner being 28; two-ness of two souls 28–30
Soul and Imagination 38–9
Soul and Soulmaking 38
Soul Connection 28–30
Soul Crisis 25, 26, 31
soul experience 28
Soulfulness: The Marriage of Shamanic and Contemporary Psychology (England) 18
soulmaking 25–7, 189; deepening of soul 25–7, 76; expanding of spirit 25–7, 76
spirit 23, 25–8, 36, 62, 71
Sri Ramakrishna 145
Steinem, Gloria 4
Stories State Existential Dilemmas 40–2
The Story as Container 43–4
Story Museum 217
storytelling: healing power 7–9; living tradition 6–7; traditional 6
Storytelling as a Healing Art 1, 6, 9, 38–46, 180; A New Gestalt: A New Way of Experiencing Ourselves 39; Reality and

Imagination 39–40; The Resonance of a Story 42–3; The Sin Against the Imagination 39; Soul and Imagination 38–9; Soul and Soulmaking 38; Stories State Existential Dilemmas 40–2; The Story as Container 43–4; Therapeutic Storywriting: Writing One's Own Story 44–6
Storytelling with Children 10, 15–6, 207–36; The Creative Power of Storytelling With Children 208–10; *The Crystal Ball* 15–6, 223–6; *Getting Rid of the Mice* 15, 214–5; *The Golden Bowl* 15, 218–9; *The Greatest Gift* 16, 231–3; *The Hat Seller* 15, 216–7; *The Naming of Cuchullin* 16, 234–6; *Pinonçita, The Very Little Girl* 15, 220–2; *The Three Spinners* 15, 211–3; *The Well of the World's End* 16, 227–30
survival self 32, 66
SwiftDeer Reagan, Harley 19, 22, 23

Tales of Soul 10, 13–4, 43, 154–90; *The Feeling In Her Bones* 14, 177–80; *The Horse of Power* 14, 163–9; *The Juniper Tree* 14, 181–5; *Saint Corentin and the Golden Fish* 14, 186–90; *Sir Gawain and the Loathly Lady* 14, 170–5; Telling Tales 176; *Vasilisa and Baba Yaga* 13–4, 155–62
Telling Tales 176
Tess of the d'Urbervilles: A Pure Woman (Hardy) 44
therapeutic storytelling 6
Therapeutic Storywriting: Writing One's Own Story (Waters) 44–6
The Three Golden Hairs 13, 134–5
The Three Princes and the Princess Nouronnihar 233
The Three Spinners 15, 211–3
Tiddalik the Frog: In the Dreamtime 13, 136–8
The Tiger and the Strawberry 13, 143–4
traditional storytelling 6
traditional tale 7
transpersonal consciousness and will 33–5
Transpersonal Tales 10, 12–3, 121, 131–53; *Dream Dilemma* 12, 133; *Iris—Rainbow Goddess* 13, 141–2; *The King and the Oak* 13, 139–40; *My Lord Bag of Rice* 13, 146–50; psychological reflections 132; *The Three Golden Hairs* 13, 134–5; *Tiddalik the Frog: In the Dreamtime* 13, 136–8; *The Tiger and the Strawberry* 13, 143–4; *A Woman Made of Salt: A Traditional Spiritual Story* 13, 145; *The Young Man, the Lion, and the Yellow-Flowered Storm-Cloud Tree* 13, 151–3
Traveller's Tales 10, 191
tri-focal vision 35
The Triphasic Model of Psychospiritual Enfoldment (Evans) 30
two-ness of two souls 28–30

UK Office for National Statistics 65
The Unsworth Dragon 12, 93–7, *96*
The Uses of Enchantment (Bettelheim) 3, 40

Variorum Shakespeare (Malone) 105
Vasilisa and Baba Yaga 13–4, 43, 155–62

Waters, Trisha 44, 45
The Well of the World's End 16, 227–30
Westwood, Jennifer 105
We've Been Eaten 45–6
What I Mean by 'Soul' 18
Wikipedia 7
'Witches' 129–30
The Witches of Windsor 12, 122–7
A Woman Made of Salt: A Traditional Spiritual Story 13, 145
The Woman Who Had Two 89
A Woman Who Is Not Owned 43
Woollard, Alan 208

The Young Man, the Lion, and the Yellow-Flowered Storm-Cloud Tree 13, 151–3

Zhuangzi 133

For Product Safety Concerns and Information please contact our EU
representative GPSR@taylorandfrancis.com
Taylor & Francis Verlag GmbH, Kaufingerstraße 24, 80331 München, Germany

www.ingramcontent.com/pod-product-compliance
Ingram Content Group UK Ltd.
Pitfield, Milton Keynes, MK11 3LW, UK
UKHW020147200926
475702UK00016B/2587

* 9 7 8 1 0 4 1 1 9 5 6 8 9 *